# Strength
# Renewed

# Strength Renewed

MEDITATIONS

*for* Your Journey *through* Breast Cancer

# Shirley Corder

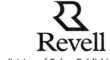

Revell

*a division of Baker Publishing Group*
Grand Rapids, Michigan

© 2012 by Shirley Corder

Published by Revell
a division of Baker Publishing Group
P.O. Box 6287, Grand Rapids, MI 49516-6287
www.revellbooks.com

Printed in the United States of America

Library of Congress Cataloging-in-Publication Data
Corder, Shirley.
    Strength renewed : meditations for your journey through breast cancer / Shirley Corder.
        p.   cm.
    Includes bibliographical references (p.    ).
    ISBN 978-0-8007-2023-0 (pbk.)
    1. Breast—Cancer—Patients—Religious life. 2. Breast—Cancer—Religious aspects—Christianity—Meditations. I. Title.
BV4910.33.C67  2012
242'.4—dc23                                                        2012010614

Unless otherwise indicated Scripture quotations are from the Holy Bible, New International Version®. NIV®. Copyright © 1973, 1978, 1984, 2011 by Biblica, Inc.™ Used by permission of Zondervan. All rights reserved worldwide. www.zondervan.com

Scripture quotations labeled CEV are from the Contemporary English Version © 1991, 1992, 1995 by American Bible Society. Used by permission.

Scripture quotations labeled GNT are from the Good News Translation—Second Edition. Copyright © 1992 by American Bible Society. Used by permission.

Scripture quotations labeled KJV are from the King James Version of the Bible.

Scripture quotations labeled Message are from *The Message* by Eugene H. Peterson, copyright © 1993, 1994, 1995, 2000, 2001, 2002. Used by permission of NavPress Publishing Group. All rights reserved.

12   13   14   15   16   17   18        7   6   5   4   3   2   1

To Rob, my husband and dearest friend, who never doubted I would survive my journey through the cancer valley. Thank you for your love, your encouragement, your practical help, and your unwavering faith in our heavenly Father.

# Contents

# Acknowledgments

Many people traveled through the cancer valley with me. Others have accompanied me on the road to publication. I praise God for each one.

I especially thank the following:

Family and friends too numerous to mention. You know who you are. Thank you for all your prayers and for your love shown in so many practical ways.

My medical team. Thank you all. One of you warned me that you didn't believe in fighting World War III with World War II weapons. You weren't kidding! Thank you for your perseverance, your willingness to step out of the box, and your faith in God.

Cecil "Cec" Murphey, writer extraordinaire, for your encouragement and input into my writing life over the past ten years. If it hadn't been for you, I doubt if I would ever have attended a writers' conference in the USA, and *Strength Renewed* would not have been published.

Dr. Vicki Crumpton, Executive Editor of Revell at Baker Publishing Group. Thank you for recognizing the need for this book and for being prepared to take the risk involved in publishing an overseas author.

Members of Truth Talk, my online writers' group: Yvonne Ortega, Geneva Iijima, and Wendy Marshall, thank you for your critiques and encouragement. Also thank you to Jan Kern for your help with my proposal and to Ruth Dell, Geni White, and Pam Corder for proofreading the finished manuscript.

Thank you, Ellen Tarver, for your enthusiasm and editing skills. The editorial team of Revell/Baker. Thank you for sharing my vision and producing a book I know will be a blessing to many.

I wish I could take away the pain and emotional trauma that my husband, Rob, my daughter, Debbie, and my sons, Stephen and David, had to go through during my year in the cancer valley. But I thank God for your prayers, love, and support during those twelve long months. Thank you for hanging in there and for not giving up on me.

Most of all, I say thank you to my heavenly Father, who saved me for the second time, and who is turning all things together for good—just like he promises in his Word.

# Introduction

Those who hope in the LORD will renew their strength. They will soar on wings like eagles; they will run and not grow weary, they will walk and not be faint.

Isaiah 40:31

When I received my diagnosis of cancer, I didn't know anything about eagles. I wanted to renew my strength, but how do you wait on anyone, even the Lord, when you're told you have cancer?

Over the following months, I learned much about eagles and even more about myself. I'm not naturally patient, but the eagle is, and so is the Lord. Gradually I learned what it meant to wait on him, and each time I did, he renewed my strength. *Strength Renewed* contains ninety meditations based on lessons I learned during my journey in the cancer valley.

When I was a student nurse, I studied the subject of cancer. I went on to care for patients at various stages of the disease. As a pastor's wife I knew the havoc cancer brought to the families of patients, and I often became part of the support team. I saw the destructive power of cancer and the way it seemed to devastate not only the body but often the spirit too.

I thought I understood cancer. Yet on November 10, 1997, I discovered how little I knew of the physical, emotional, and spiritual roller coaster that cancer creates. It took three short words spoken by an uncaring radiologist: "You have cancer." I'd heard those words before, but this time they were directed at me.

My first reaction to the diagnosis was to call out to the Lord. I knew I needed help from above, and I needed it right away.

I grew up in a home where my parents had a nominal belief in God. As a teenager, I attended church regularly and participated as a young musician and children's Sunday school teacher. In my late teenage years I experienced a spiritual renewal. From then on, my faith grew. By the time cancer disrupted my life, my husband and I had been in full-time Christian ministry for twenty-eight years.

I know of people who came to faith as a result of cancer, and I praise God for them. Others, like me, were already walking with the Lord when the disease made itself known. Wherever you are spiritually, my prayer is that this book will strengthen your faith. If your relationship with God is still at an intellectual level, then I trust that as you work through these meditations, God himself will ignite the sparks of faith in you. Some people survive cancer without leaning on the Lord. I couldn't have—and I don't believe you'd want to.

I also needed friends to keep me company during this difficult time, especially one friend who would walk through the experience with me. That person had to be someone who would love me no matter what I looked like, how I behaved, or what I said. He or she would have to be an encourager but also care enough to say "Enough!" and stop me from wallowing in misery. I would need someone to dry my tears, hold me close when I trembled, and rejoice over the little successes that marked my year in treatment. In short, that person had to love me unconditionally.

I didn't have to look far. My husband, Rob, stepped into the role without hesitation.

A cancer diagnosis often has adverse effects on a marriage, and sadly, many don't survive. I can understand this. The patient goes through such a wide range of emotions it's sometimes hard to recognize the person you married. Yet Rob never flinched from his role as husband, lover, and friend. He also never wavered from his faith in God and held firmly to his belief that together we would overcome this disease and life would resume some sense of normalcy.

If you are battling cancer, I pray you find such a friend. Please don't isolate yourself; instead, nurture your relationships. Allow the Lord to raise up people who will love you through this time. If you are one of those friends, I pray that as you read the meditations you will empathize with your loved one and grow in your understanding and ability to offer support.

In addition to needing a friend, I longed to meet or speak to people who had been through what I was facing and had not only survived but gone on to have a fulfilling life. Patients I once nursed had recovered and moved on to other places. Beulah, the cancer survivor who came to see me from the Reach for Recovery organization, appeared glamorous, confident, and healthy. This encouraged me, but she had only survived ten years at that point. I was fifty-two. I wanted to meet someone who'd lived much longer.

One morning I received a phone call from a lady by the name of Molly. She worked at the head office of my husband's denomination. She said, "Shirley, you can beat this. I had breast cancer thirty-five years ago, and I am still well today." Those words encouraged me more than any others during those dreadful early days of cancer. I have never met Molly, but she became my role model. If she could live thirty-five years after her diagnosis, so could I. I haven't reached the thirty-five-year mark yet, but it's been fifteen years since I heard those three dreadful words, "You have cancer."

As a result of cancer, I had to take a break from nursing, so I turned to my favorite hobby: writing. Today, I'm a published author—and I love it. If it hadn't been for cancer, I doubt this would have happened.

Years after my diagnosis, I sensed a prompt from the Lord to write this book for people struggling through the cancer valley. You may be a patient, or perhaps the disease has afflicted someone you care for. Possibly you work with someone who has cancer or you're in the medical field. Whatever your involvement, I pray the stories in this book will help you wait on the Lord.

During that long and difficult year of treatment, there were times I soared over the valley. Other times I plummeted to the depths. Yet the loving wings of my heavenly Father always came underneath me before I hit the ground and lifted me back into his presence. He'll do the same for you as you seek to draw close to him through these meditations.

*Strength Renewed* is a book of daily devotional readings that follows the cancer journey chronologically. You can, however, read the chapters in any order. Stories from my own experience link to relevant Scripture readings. Three questions follow each meditation and will help you apply the material to your own particular cancer journey. Answer the questions as honestly as you know how, whether you are a patient or a supporter. There are no right or wrong answers, for no two people are alike.

Although most of the messages and questions will be geared toward the patient, supporters should also read the material and answer the questions as best they can. Doing so will give them a clearer understanding of what the patient is going through.

Jot down your answers in a notebook and allow the words to assist you in waiting upon the Lord. He will then renew your strength and help you rise and soar as you go through your treatment period.

*But those who wait upon God get fresh strength. They spread their wings and soar like eagles, they run and don't get tired, they walk and don't lag behind.*

ISAIAH 40:31 MESSAGE

# 1

## The Clock Is Ticking

READ: *Luke 1:26-35*

Whatever Mary planned for her future, it didn't include pregnancy before marriage.

She grew up in the small town of Nazareth where everyone knew everybody. Her parents taught her to believe in the only true God, and she eagerly looked forward to the coming Messiah.

The day an angel visited her with the shattering news that she was about to become pregnant, Mary's life changed forever. Yet because of her obedience, the Messiah became part of her family tree. She became the most blessed of women—the mother of our Lord Jesus. History divided into BC and AD—"before Christ" and "anno Domini." The world would never be the same again.

On November 10, 1997, my life changed forever with the words "you have cancer." Suddenly I knew my life had an end. The days left to me were limited. Even if I conquered the mass that had invaded my breast, one day I would run out of time. Whether I suffered a massive heart attack, got run over by a drunk driver, or, God forbid, died of cancer, I only had a certain number of days left. And they were running out.

Of course, that had always been the case, but until that moment life was too full to consider my mortality. Now I could think of nothing else. *I have cancer.*

Fifteen years later, my life is divided into BC and AC: "before cancer" and "after cancer." Those three harsh words, "you have cancer," transformed my life. Yet they really made no difference as to how long I still have on earth. God already knows how many days I will live, and they aren't numbered by cancer.

- How did you react to the words "you have cancer," whether addressed to you or to someone you love?
- What, for you, is the most difficult part of this diagnosis?
- As you look ahead, what sort of future do you visualize AC ("after cancer")?

Your cancer diagnosis didn't take God by surprise. He isn't confused about what to do. Right now, stretch out your hand. Allow him to take hold of it and walk with you into the future. Yes, your life's clock is ticking—but you know what? God made the clock.

**LET'S PRAY:** Lord God, you know how scared I am. Help me to trust you and to remember that you made this body of mine—and you don't make mistakes. Please give me your peace and help me remember that you, and you alone, know how many days I have left. Amen.

*Did you not . . . clothe me with skin and flesh and knit me together with bones and sinews?*

JOB 10:10–11

# 2

## Search for Peace

READ: *Psalm 46:1–11*

Y ou have cancer." How was this possible? There was no history of breast cancer in my family. I ate a healthy diet and looked well. I held down a full-time job and participated in many church activities. How could I have a life-threatening illness? Besides, cancer happened to other people, not me.

"Oh Lord," I whispered. "Where are you? How can this be true?" My mind raced as I tried to grasp the news I'd just heard. How I wished I could undo the last hour and step back in time.

Psalm 46 assures us that even if the earth is shaken and the mountains fall into the sea, God will still be there as our shelter and strength. He will always be ready to help in times of trouble.

My earth had certainly been shaken. I searched for assurance that God was still close by, that he would be my shelter and strength. I walked across the parking lot on my way to the car. On my way home. On my way to break the news to my husband . . .

High above my head, wisps of cloud drifted across the African sky, nudged by a breeze I couldn't feel down on earth. A tiny image of a plane soared noiselessly across the blue. The warmth of the sun seeped into my body and brought with it a feeling of calm. Somewhere in the depths of my body, beyond the reach of ultrasound, God was at work. I didn't understand how I could have cancer, but God knew, and he was still in control. I had to believe that.

- What are some of the ways cancer has shaken your life?
- How did you hear the diagnosis of cancer? Do you believe God was with you at that time?
- In hindsight, can you think of any one thing God has done to prepare you for this challenge?

Cancer may have blindsided you like it did me, but it didn't take God by surprise. He saw it coming, and he promises to be your shelter and strength.

**LET'S PRAY:** Loving Father, I don't know why this happened, but I have to believe you're still in control. Help me to grow closer to you through this time. Please grant me your peace. Amen.

*Jesus said, "Peace I leave with you; my peace I give you. I do not give to you as the world gives. Do not let your hearts be troubled and do not be afraid."*

JOHN 14:27

# 3

# It's Not Easy

**READ:** *James 3:3-6*

It didn't take me long to learn there's no easy way to break the news of cancer. I tried rehearsing different approaches, but it always ended up the same: "I have cancer."

People responded in different ways. My husband looked aghast and then took me in his arms. When I phoned Stephen, the older of our two sons, his initial reaction was silence. Then he reminded me that God was in control, not medical science. David, our youngest, swallowed hard, then pulled me out of my chair and enveloped me in a comforting hug. My elderly mother took a deep breath and went into battle for me.

Family members, friends, or mere acquaintances all shared one reaction: shock. No matter how they tried to hide it, I always saw a look of horror flash across their faces.

Some immediately tried to reassure me. Others sought *my* reassurance that I'd survive. A number asked me questions, often before I knew the answers myself. Still others launched into pep talks or quoted Scripture at me. Several even saw the need to tell me about someone else they knew who had cancer. Two things soon became clear: I couldn't find an easy way to tell them, and they had no idea how to respond.

In his letter to the early church, James compares the tongue to the rudder of a ship. He points out that a small rudder can steer a big ship (3:4). I didn't know how to break the news, but I prayed that the Lord would guide my words.

- How do you tell people about your cancer diagnosis?
- What has been the most encouraging response?
- In what ways has the news impacted those closest to you?

When one person gets cancer, the whole family gets cancer. Thank the Lord now for those who will stand by you through this time. They need your prayers—and your understanding.

**LET'S PRAY:** Lord, I hate having to tell my family this news. There doesn't seem to be an easy way to say it, so please give me the best words for each person. Give them the strength they will need over the coming weeks. Please draw us close during this anxious time. Amen.

*[Love] always protects, always trusts, always hopes, always perseveres.*

1 CORINTHIANS 13:7

# 4

## I Wasn't Born Brave

READ: *Joshua 1:1-9*

I always imagined Joshua to be a strong and capable leader, a brave and fearless warrior. After Moses died, God chose Joshua to lead the children of Israel. He brought them to the Jordan River. After they crossed it they would at last take possession of the Promised Land. It is interesting that not once, not twice, but three times in the first nine verses of the book of Joshua, God commands the new Israelite commander to have courage, to not be afraid. Why would he do that if Joshua was the tough man of war I thought him to be?

Joshua wasn't born brave. He needed a lot of encouragement. As he stepped out in faith, he had to make a conscious decision to not be afraid. He chose to step with courage and dignity into the frightening situation God had opened for him. God knew this man's potential, yet Joshua was terrified.

I wasn't born brave either. In the few days between the mammogram and my surgery, I alternated between feelings of calm and dread. The odds of my surviving to old age seemed poor. The surgeon warned I would almost certainly need radiation. It had never occurred to me there might be more than surgery. I planned to go back to work as soon as my stitches were removed, but for how long would I be able to work? Would I be badly disfigured by the surgery? Would the cancer ultimately destroy me?

The words of the radiologist kept ringing in my ears: "I doubt if they'll be able to get it all out."

I had a good surgeon—but would he be good enough? Would my body cope with the demands of surgery and radiation? Several times a day my mind whimpered, "I'm afraid. This is too much for me." Each time I sensed God saying, "Don't be afraid. Have courage. I'm here. I won't let you down."

- What is your greatest fear?
- How do you think God might respond to your fears?
- Can you think of a verse in Scripture that will give you courage to move forward? Look it up now.

Make no mistake, a cancer diagnosis is a living nightmare. Stepping toward the surgery and into the unknown is terrifying and requires great courage. It's okay to be scared. God is not disappointed by your fear. He doesn't scold you for your reluctance to move on.

**LET'S PRAY:** Lord God, you know my fears. You understand how overwhelming life seems at the moment. Help me to keep my eyes on you. I want to face the future with courage and dignity. Stay real close, Lord, please. Amen.

*In God I trust and am not afraid. What can man do to me?*

PSALM 56:11

# 5

# In Need of a Miracle

READ: *Acts 3:1–8*

As the news got out about my cancer, it became difficult to remain positive. As a nurse and a pastor's wife, I knew of many who had lost their battle with cancer. I had watched others in whom the disease continued to advance no matter what treatment they went through. No hope. No future.

Well-meaning folks told me to trust God for a supernatural miracle of healing. That made me uneasy. Did they mean I shouldn't trust the doctors? Did they want me to refuse medical intervention and expect God to heal me without conservative treatment? Others urged me to follow through with the surgery and any further treatment and trust God to work through the doctors. Should I continue treatment, or should I trust God for an outright miracle?

The crippled man in Acts 3 was en route to his usual location—a spot near the so-called Beautiful Gate. Every day his friends placed him near this temple entrance so he could beg for a living. Lame from birth, the man was beyond medical help. The situation could only deteriorate as he grew older. He looked around at other crippled men and could see the way his life would end. No hope. No joy. No sense of anticipation.

As the small group drew near to the gate, the beggar spotted two men on their way into the temple. He called to them in hopes of a handout. Instead, they instructed him to pay attention.

"I don't have any money," Peter said, "but I'll give you what I have."

The man probably looked at them with a flicker of hope. Would they give him clothing? Food? Anything would help his miserable existence.

Instead, Peter reached out, grasped his right hand, and heaved him to his feet. The man's ankles strengthened, and for the first time in his life he could walk.

When I read this passage, I knew I should ask the Lord for a miracle but continue with the medical plans. The Lord would heal me in his way and in his time. I just needed to trust.

- What decisions confuse you at the moment?
- Whom can you speak to about those decisions?
- Why not ask the Lord now for a miracle?

Forget the future and focus on the present. Tell God how you feel, and don't be afraid to ask him for a miracle. But don't forget, he can also work a miracle through your doctors—he created medical science.

**LET'S PRAY:** Lord, thank you that you're in control of my future. Help me to trust you, and please grant me a miracle of healing in your time and in your way. Amen.

*So if the Son sets you free, you will be free indeed.*

JOHN 8:36

# 6

## Let's Be Real

READ: *John 9:1-11*

Jesus and his disicples came across a man who had been blind all his life.

"Who's to blame for this man's blindness?" the disciples asked Jesus.

"No one," Jesus replied. He explained that God's power would be revealed as a result of the man's disability.

I have no idea why I got breast cancer. In my family I have the dubious honor of being the first and, at the time of this writing, the only one ever to have the disease. When people heard of my diagnosis, one of their first questions was often, "Is it in your family?" In other words, "Who's to blame?"

I had often heard cancer referred to as "the Big C" or simply "CA." Now I wondered why people didn't want to call it by its name. Was it their way of coping with the disease, a form of denial? Or were they for some reason ashamed or embarrassed by their diagnosis? After all, if you get the flu you don't mind telling people. So why should I be ashamed of having cancer? I hadn't done anything shameful to cause rogue cells to form the malignant tumor. Yet visitors also avoided the word *cancer*. They spoke of my "illness" or my "problem." They encouraged me to fight "it" and to believe the Lord could help me overcome the "challenge."

From the outset I decided to be open about my diagnosis. I had cancer. I didn't understand why God allowed me to get this dreaded disease, but he had. And according to his Word, *all things* would work together for good because I loved him (Rom. 8:28). I had to believe "all things" included cancer. If I didn't accept that, I would be saying my diagnosis was beyond God's control. And I knew it wasn't.

So I determined to remain as upbeat as possible, learn as much as I could, and be open about my disease. I had cancer. It wasn't my fault, and I had no one else to blame. Somehow God would use it for good. I had to believe that.

- How do you refer to your cancer? Do you call it by its name?
- Are you able to trust God with your future, or do you struggle with this concept?
- What does it mean to you that "in all things" God is at work in your situation?

It's important to face your diagnosis. When you call cancer by any other name, it becomes more difficult to come to terms with an already tough situation. Cancer is finite. God is way bigger.

**LET'S PRAY:** Lord, I don't understand why you've allowed me to get cancer, but you have. I want to believe you're going to use this in a good way, so please help me to speak openly about it. Use my openness to bless others, I pray. Amen.

*In all things God works for the good of those who love him, who have been called according to his purpose.*

ROMANS 8:28

# 7

# Who's to Blame?

READ: *Philemon 1-10*

Well-meaning people made suggestions as to why I developed cancer. Some blamed my food, although I ate a healthier diet than most. Others suggested soil contamination. There wasn't much I could do about that. Anyway, everyone ate vegetables from the same soil. Several people thought it was because I didn't breast-feed my babies. While that is believed to be one of many possible contributing causes, not everyone who bottle-feeds their babies gets breast cancer. So why did I?

Could I really blame the food my parents fed me as a child? Could I have avoided cancer by doing something different? Whose fault was it? No matter the cause, it had happened. Nothing would reverse the diagnosis.

The book of Philemon was written by Paul when he was under house arrest. Although he was able to receive visitors, Romans guarded Paul around the clock and he was not allowed to leave home. Nevertheless, he continued to lead others to Christ and encouraged the young churches with his writings.

At least Paul knew why he was in custody. His open preaching and involvement with the Christian church brought about his arrest. Yet as he dug deeper for understanding, he remembered the Lord's words: "Just as you have told others about me in Jerusalem, you must also tell about me in Rome" (Acts 23:11 CEV).

Paul saw his incarceration as part of the Lord's plan to extend the kingdom. As a result of his imprisonment, he now lived in

Rome. He had ample opportunity to teach about Jesus and led a number of people into the Christian faith (Philem. 7).

Despite his difficult circumstances, Paul believed that Christ was in control. He believed God could use him even while under house arrest. Instead of lamenting his misfortunes, he continued to encourage others.

- Can you see any ways Jesus might use your cancer to bless others?
- Is Christ really in control of your circumstances? If so, what does it mean to you?
- Is there someone you can encourage today?

I didn't know why I had cancer, but as I read about Paul, I asked, "Is it possible that I am right where the Lord wants me to be? Does he want to use my circumstances to reach out to others?" These were not easy questions, but as I worked through them, I found myself looking for ways to use my circumstances for good.

**LET'S PRAY:** Lord Jesus, I grapple with why I have cancer. Help me to accept that whatever the reasons may be, you are able to bless me. Please also bless others through me. Help me to get my eyes off my suffering and to rejoice in your love. Amen.

*For our light and momentary troubles are achieving for us an eternal glory that far outweighs them all.*

2 CORINTHIANS 4:17

# 8

# Role Reversal

READ: *Matthew 26:36–43*

I once read an article about the role reversal that takes place between parents and their adult children. As the parents become frail and decision-making becomes difficult, the children have to step in and help guide them. The children often have to parent their parents.

When I faced cancer treatment, my mother was my only parent still alive. Despite her fierce independence, encroaching blindness caused her to need my help more and more. That was to be expected; she was elderly and almost totally blind.

But I was in my early fifties when cancer hit me. Many people made decisions on my behalf. Doctors, medical technicians, my husband, even our oldest son took over in situations where normally I would have determined the next move. I didn't like having to be dependent on others one bit.

I'm sure Jesus didn't like it either.

For three years, he had led his disciples, taught them about God, and supported them in every possible way. Now the roles were reversed. He needed them—and the disciples didn't do very well. When he took three of them to one side and asked them to pray for him, they fell asleep. When the soldiers came to arrest him, Peter lopped off someone's ear. After Jesus replaced the ear, the disciples all fled.

- What relationship, if any, has changed for you since your cancer diagnosis?
- How good are you at accepting help from others, especially those whom you normally lead?
- Are there people who would like to do things for you if you would allow them to?

It is never easy to admit you need assistance. Yet if a person helps you in a gracious way, the Bible says it's as if they are doing it unto the Lord (see Matt. 25:37–40). By not allowing others to help us, are we perhaps robbing them of blessings?

**LET'S PRAY:** Lord God, thank you for those who want to help me during this difficult time. Thank you too for those who would like to do more if I let them. Forgive me if I have prevented them by my independence. Help me to appreciate and accept assistance where it's needed. Amen.

*The King will reply, "Truly I tell you, whatever you did for one of the least of these brothers and sisters of mine, you did for me."*

MATTHEW 25:40

# 9

# A Secret Weapon

READ: *Habakkuk 3:17-19*

Habakkuk's message of praise was not new to me. For years Rob and I had taught on the subjects of praise and worship. We often pointed out how, if we praise God when things are tough, we show our trust in him. By praising God in all things, we open the way for him to work in our lives.

Yada yada yada. It all sounded so correct, so theological, so . . . easy. Did "all things" really include cancer?

As the day of my surgery approached, I remembered Paul's instruction to "give thanks in all circumstances" (1 Thess. 5:18). How I struggled to put this into practice!

I praised even though I didn't feel like it. I thanked the Lord that my body was in good condition and that I would cope well with the operation. I praised him that the cancer had been found now and not a year from now when it definitely would have been too late.

I gave thanks for the surgeon, whom I didn't like at first but grew to respect. I praised the Lord for whatever lessons he would teach me throughout this whole experience. As I gave thanks, my attitude underwent a shift. I grew stronger in my belief that God would bring me through this time. Somehow he would use this unwanted development for good. He had to. He promised in his Word.

The beauty of having praise as a weapon is that no one needed to know when I used it. When people made thoughtless comments, I silently thanked the Lord that they were wrong. If I felt fear, I quickly shot up a prayer of "Help Lord! I'm praising you here!"

I praised the Lord that he knew what the surgeon would find. I praised God that he would ensure the surgeon got it all out. Praise the Lord in *all* situations? More often than not, I didn't feel in the least thankful. But God said "praise!" and so praise I did. Most of the time.

- What's easier, to praise the Lord or to panic?
- Can you think of one thing you can be grateful for about *your* cancer, and thank the Lord for that now?
- In what way can you praise God today, even if you don't feel like it?

Nothing in Scripture says you have to *feel* your praise. Don't worry if your words feel insincere. Prayer is a weapon. The more you praise, the easier it will become.

**LET'S PRAY:** Lord God, you say I should give thanks to you in all things. I guess that means cancer too. So I praise you for the surgery and for the treatment that I dread. You know I don't really mean these words right now, but I use the weapon of praise in faith—and I trust you to take control. Amen.

*I praise your promises! I trust you and am not afraid. No one can harm me.*

PSALM 56:4 CEV

# 10

## The Writing on My Hands

READ: *Psalm 139:13-18*

W hy do you always write on your hands?" an irritated gentleman once asked me. "Here's a piece of paper."

"No, thanks," I replied. "I'm likely to lose the paper. I won't lose my hand."

Writing on my hand has been a habit of mine for years. Whenever I hear a snippet of information I need to remember until I get home, I quickly jot a couple of words on the palm of my hand. When I get home and notice the writing, I know it's important. On a few occasions I forget and wash my hands. Then I panic to remember what I wrote.

One morning I read Psalm 139 and saw God had been present in my life since before my conception. He watched over me as I grew in my mother's womb. He was there at my birth and throughout my childhood. I'm sure I brought sorrow to my heavenly Father many times, yet his love for me never wavered.

The angels rejoiced with God the night I committed my life to him, changing me forever. What's more, Isaiah 49:16 says he engraved my name on the palms of his hands.

So what went wrong? Why did I get cancer? Did God wash his hands? Did he forget about me? Did eternity stop for a moment while he tried to remember what he'd written there?

God knew I had cancer long before the mammogram revealed its presence. He'd seen those first cells divide in my breast and begin their abnormal growth. He watched the tumor grow, and he saw it start to spread. Yet he never forgot about me. He couldn't. You see, he didn't *write* my name on his palm. He engraved it. He can't wash it away. I am too important to him.

- How does it make you feel, knowing that God was aware you had cancer before you even knew?
- Why would God engrave *your* name on his hand?
- What difference does it make to know God will never forget you?

It's hard to understand how a loving God could allow cancer to develop in one of his children and not stop it. Nor do I understand why we are so important to him, but I'm glad we are. I know he hasn't forgotten me—or you. He never will.

**LET'S PRAY:** Lord, I don't understand how you can love me so much and yet let me get cancer. Nor do I understand why I'm important to you. Nevertheless, thank you that you know me by name and will never forget me. I trust you, even when I don't understand. Amen.

*See, I have engraved you on the palms of my hands.*

ISAIAH 49:16

# 11

# Please Pray for Me

READ: *Mark 5:25-34*

Many stories in Scripture tell of God's healing power. Just a few examples are the woman with the bleeding problem, several men who were born blind or crippled, and Jairus's daughter. I personally knew people who had been miraculously healed, and in our own family we'd seen the Lord intervene in amazing ways. He could heal others; he could heal me too.

As I told family and friends of my diagnosis, they were all shocked, but each one reacted differently. Everyone except my youngest son was taken by surprise. (For some reason, God told David that morning that I had cancer, before I even knew.) After recovering from the shock, most of the family expressed confidence that I would be fine after the surgery and went out of their way to reassure me.

Many said they would pray for me and they'd get others to pray. Yet not one, apart from Rob, prayed *with* me. And no one suggested the Lord might heal me. I found that strange and scary.

The day before my scheduled surgery, which was a Sunday, the elders and leaders anointed me with oil after our church service. They prayed for strength for Rob and for guidance for the surgeon. They prayed for wisdom if any decisions needed to be made with regard to other treatment. Then at last one person prayed for me— that I would have peace. No one prayed that God would heal me. They prayed for peace.

- Has someone prayed with you for healing? If not, whom can you ask?
- Is it possible your healing may involve more than surgery?
- In what way are you praying for your own healing?

Sometimes people are healed instantly. More often, healing takes time and even treatment. And sometimes we receive the ultimate healing—when the Lord takes us to be with him. God promises to hear and answer our prayers, but he doesn't always answer the way we want him to.

**LET'S PRAY:** Lord, I don't want to go through this. *Cancer* is such a scary word. Yet I put my trust in you now. Hold me close and never let me go. Amen.

*Do not be anxious about anything, but in every situation, by prayer and petition, with thanksgiving, present your requests to God.*

PHILIPPIANS 4:6

# 12

# My True Value

READ: *Isaiah 43:1-7*

I hunted everywhere for the missing fifty rand* note. I couldn't find it anywhere. Several days later it turned up—in the ironing. Folded neatly, it had been tucked in the pocket of my slacks when I threw them into the washing machine. Washed, spun, and hung out to dry, it was no longer "filthy lucre." The crisp, well-laundered note was intact, and I could use it for my groceries. Although it looked like a new note, its cleanliness didn't increase its value. For that matter, if it had come apart in the wash it would still have been worth R50.

There's a strange thing about a cancer diagnosis. If I had broken my leg or been rushed to the hospital for an emergency appendectomy, people would have sympathized and anticipated me back in circulation within a few weeks. Yet when I told people I had cancer, they were clearly taken aback. I felt as if I'd let them down. It was as if the diagnosis of cancer had depreciated my value.

In the book of Isaiah, God says this of his people: "I will give up whole nations to save your life, because you are precious to me and because I love you and give you honor" (Isa. 43:4 GNT).

No matter how serious my cancer, no matter what treatment I faced, nothing would ever separate me from God. And my value would never depreciate. As the psalmist says, "I am fearfully and wonderfully made; [God's] works are wonderful" (Ps. 139:14).

*The rand (ZAR or R) is the unit of currency in South Africa.

- Why do you think *you* are valuable to God?
- How much does your heavenly Father value you? Ask him to show you.
- According to the above Scriptures, what can depreciate your value in God's sight?

How good to know that my value in God's sight does not depend on my looks. It doesn't matter how much hair I have, how stable my emotions are, or how much food I keep down. God loves me with an everlasting love—and I am valuable in his sight.

**LET'S PRAY:** Lord, how good it is to know that no matter what effects cancer or treatment may have on me, you value me. Thank you that I am precious in your sight. Amen.

*When you are in trouble, call out to me. I will answer and be there to protect and honor you.*

PSALM 91:15 CEV

# 13

# You Still There, Lord?

READ: *1 Peter 1:3-9*

I'd made many mistakes in my life. I'd been disobedient to God. I'd questioned his wisdom. But since the day Christ became a reality in my life, I had attempted to live close to God. I didn't ask for special favors from him, but I certainly didn't expect him to allow me to get cancer.

"Why you?" a number of friends asked me. "Of all people, why should you go through this?"

"Why not me?" I would reply. "At least I know the Lord. If I die, I know where I'm going."

I never doubted this, but many times I wished he would *show* me why. If his Word was true, and I believed it was, God wouldn't allow me to suffer more than I could cope with. I admit, there were times I wanted to remind him of my limitations. Nevertheless, I had to believe he would bring me through the ordeal of cancer and deliver me whole at the end.

Job went through a far worse time than I did. He lost most of his family and possessions. Festering sores covered his body. Even his wife turned from him. "Curse God and die," she advised. His friends turned out to be self-righteous snobs with no empathy.

Throughout that dreadful time, Job saw no sign of God's love and compassion. His life was a mess. Every aspect of it seemed to have fallen apart. The tortured man examined his life and searched for where he'd gone wrong. Sure, he'd been disobedient at times. He'd questioned God's wisdom and even cursed the day of his birth. Yet he'd attempted to live close to God. After all he went through, Job arrived at the conclusion: "God knows every step I take." Job only had to believe. So did I.

I *had* to believe God was still in control. If I didn't, that meant Satan was stronger than God. I couldn't live with that.

- What is the worst thing you're dealing with right now?
- Whom can you speak to who will encourage you in your faith?
- Can you think of one good thing God might bring out of this? Just one?

I didn't understand why I had to go through this, but I believed it would somehow fit into God's plan for my life. I tried to hold on to the thought, "Good *will* come from this." My life would be richer for the experience.

Where was God? Even when I couldn't sense his presence, I had to believe he was right there with me.

**LET'S PRAY:** Lord, I hate what's happening to me right now. I look forward to the time when I see the blessings you bring out of this. Please reassure me of your presence and your love. Amen.

*But he knows the way that I take; when he has tested me, I will come forth as gold.*

JOB 23:10

# 14

## Are You Not God?

READMatthew 16:13-17*

I lay in bed and tried to pray. My husband snored softly next to me. "Lord, speak to me," I pleaded. "Tell me you're in control."

I read of a family who had a time of prayer based on 2 Chronicles 20:6 (below). One of them prayed, "Are you not the God in heaven?" Another family member followed with, "Are you not the God who sealed the mouths of lions and spared Daniel?" Then another added, "Are you not the God who fed five thousand people with a few small fish and loaves?" And so they continued.

I whispered into the dark, "Are you not the God who created me?" I continued, "Are you not the God who watched over me as I was being formed in my mother's womb?" He knew the cancer was there before the ultrasound picked it up.

"Are you not the God who prompted me to insist on a mammogram even when the doctor didn't want me to have one?" He had brought me safely to this place.

"Are you not the God who gave me a husband and family to stand with me during this time?" I felt my faith grow as I continued. I longed to wake my husband and get him involved.

"Are you not the God who goes into surgery ahead of me tomorrow?" My spirits lifted as I added, "Are you not the God who will guide the surgeon as he operates?"

I curled onto my side and closed my eyes. "And are you not the God who will help me sleep until morning and wake refreshed?"

The sleeping pill the doctor had insisted I take kicked in. I slipped into a peaceful sleep and didn't wake until the alarm rang.

- How will you complete the question: "Are you not the God who . . . ?"
- Why not take a few minutes to ask him the question at least once? Try to come up with others.
- What difference does it make to you to realize that he *is* that God?

As we focus our prayers on how powerful and all-seeing our God is, our problems become more manageable. He *is* the God in heaven who rules over this earth. He *is* the God who watches over my life—and yours. He *is* the God no one, nothing—not even cancer—can withstand.

**LET'S PRAY:** Lord, are you not the God who walks ahead of me into the future? Thank you for that assurance. Help me never to forget you're right there in front of me. Amen.

*Lord, the God of our ancestors, are you not the God who is in heaven? . . . Power and might are in your hand, and no one can withstand you.*

2 CHRONICLES 20:6

# 15

# A Win-Win Situation

READ: *John 11:17–27*

**B**efore Jesus raised Lazarus from the dead, he said to Martha, "Whoever lives by believing in me will never die." He then asked Martha a challenging question: "Do you believe this?" (John 11:26).

I imagine Martha took a deep breath before she answered. Did she believe this? Do you? Do I?

Jesus gave Lazarus his life back for a time, but Lazarus was mortal and eventually he died again. Yet before Lazarus died the second time, Jesus died on the cross. He gave up his physical life to make it possible for all those who believe in God to have eternal life.

The well-known Scripture says, "God loved the world so much that he gave his only Son, so that everyone who believes in him may not die but have eternal life" (John 3:16 GNT). I believed in Jesus, so I knew I had eternal life. However, at that point of my cancer struggle I wanted physical life too. I wasn't ready to move on from my earthly body. I longed for more time on earth.

God answered my prayer, and I've had fifteen years of good health following my cancer diagnosis.

- Jesus died for *you*. What does that mean to you personally?
- When you die, whenever that may be, are you certain you will go to be with God in heaven?*

*If not, please read "New Relationship" on p. 192.

- What plans do you have for your future here on earth, however long that may be?

It is easy to believe in eternal life when we're healthy. When we're faced with our own mortality, it's not so easy. Paul sums up our situation this way: "To live is Christ and to die is gain" (Phil. 1:21). If we live, we'll be guided and encouraged by the Lord. If we die physically, we will be in his presence, away from the challenges of life here on earth. It's a win-win situation.

**LET'S PRAY:** Lord God, salvation is an amazing gift. Thank you that I don't need to fear death. Thank you that when the time comes, I will go to live with you for eternity. Amen.

*If we live, we live for the Lord; and if we die, we die for the Lord. So, whether we live or die, we belong to the Lord.*

ROMANS 14:8

# 16

## Joy? Now?

READ: *1 Corinthians 1:25-28*

The night before surgery, my husband and I curled up together in bed. Fear threatened to choke me. Could this be real? Would I survive the surgery? What if they opened me and just closed me again, unable to remove all the cancer? My thoughts went wild as I imagined the worst scenario.

To my surprise, following the spiritual exercise I described earlier ("Are You Not God?" p. 40), I slept better than normal and awoke bright and cheerful. When I arrived at the hospital, an onlooker would have thought I was going to visit a friend who had undergone a minor procedure. I walked with a spring in my step and chuckled with my husband as I commented that when I walked back out of this same building I would be a different person.

In Paul's first letter to the Corinthians, he reminds us that often the wisdom of man is foolishness to God. In the same way, the wisdom of God makes no sense to the world.

On a number of occasions during my stay in the hospital I experienced this same joy. I often laughed with visitors and cracked jokes to the other patients, despite a degree of pain and discomfort and a gloomy prognosis. My joy was not normal—it could only have come from the Lord.

- When, if ever, have you experienced a feeling of calm or joy that didn't make sense?

- What area of foolishness in your life could perhaps be part of God's wisdom?
- When was the last time you laughed out loud? Do you need to ask the Lord to increase your joy?

Throughout the year, I went through some tough times and often felt as if I'd never smile again. Yet a short time later, I'd see the funny side of the situation and make a joke. Some found this strange—and perhaps they were right. I'm sure many times visitors or nursing staff thought I was putting on an act. My attitude often didn't make sense, but the joy was real. It came from God, and how I appreciated those occasions.

**LET'S PRAY:** Lord, thank you that what doesn't make sense to the world may well be part of your wisdom. Thank you for the times when I have a peace or joy that doesn't make human sense. Help me to ask for your joy and anticipate it. Amen.

*The joy of the LORD is your strength.*

NEHEMIAH 8:10

# 17

# The Bigger Plan

READ: *Genesis 45:3-8*

The reality of my cancer diagnosis only set in after surgery. Until then, it had seemed more like a bad story with no ending. As I lay awake during the long night hours, I realized that God had known all about the cancer growing inside my body. So why hadn't he stopped it?

In the story of Joseph, we read how this brash young man antagonized his brothers with his boastful attitude and words. Eventually they'd had enough, and they sold him into slavery.

Joseph ended up in Egypt, far from home, alone and frightened. He went through some dark times of suffering. Many times he must have wondered, "Why? What did I do to deserve this?"

When Joseph was thirty, Pharaoh appointed him his second-in-command. During a seven-year period of rich harvest, Joseph got the country to store a huge quantity of grain. When famine struck the land, Egypt had sufficient food to meet not only their own needs but also to help foreigners who came looking to buy grain.

One day Joseph's brothers came to ask the Pharaoh for food. To their amazement and terror, they discovered the person in charge was none other than their long-lost brother, Joseph.

The story had all the makings of a tragedy, but Joseph had come to accept God's sovereignty in his life. He realized that although his brothers had meant him harm, God had kept him safe. God used the brothers' wicked actions to get Joseph where he wanted him.

My cancer story also had the makings of a tragedy, yet God kept me safe too. The devil sought to destroy me and discredit my testimony. But God wanted me where I would testify to others about his saving power. Did God cause my cancer? No, I don't believe he did. He didn't throw Joseph into the pit or sell him to slave traders either. But he sure used the result.

- How do you feel toward God for allowing your cancer?
- What makes it seem as if cancer has taken over your life?
- In what way has God helped you cope with your present circumstances?

It's been fifteen years since my cancer diagnosis. If it hadn't been for that horrible time, I would never have written this book. I would never have been able to come alongside other cancer victims and support them through their tough times of treatment. God wouldn't have used me to help cancer victims across the world via the internet. Even though I didn't always feel that he did, my Father had everything under control.

**LET'S PRAY:** Father, forgive me for sometimes being angry with you or for resenting others. Help me to remember your promise to work out all things for good. Amen.

*When times are good, be happy; but when times are bad, consider this: God has made the one as well as the other.*

ECCLESIASTES 7:14

# 18

# A Lion-Sized Gift

READ: *Psalm 139:1-6*

The first night after my surgery, Stephen, my older son, walked into the ward. Through my drug-induced haze, I glimpsed a magnificent arrangement of pink roses. "Thank you so much," I mumbled. Then he presented me with a small stuffed lion. He explained he had seen it on the counter of the shop where he bought me a get-well card and felt compelled to buy it for me. I thought this was strange. I had never been a cuddly toy type of person. Stephen put it on my bedside locker, and I forgot it.

Later that night, alone and in pain, I noticed the little lion on the locker and reached for it. Right then, I had no one else to hold on to. No one else to soak up my tears. No one else to comfort me. I pulled him close and tucked him under my cheek. That little lion, or Squiffles as I named him, gave me something to hang on to and cuddle until the drugs took effect and I drifted back to sleep.

Without a doubt, God prompted Stephen to buy me that lion. God knew I would need something soft and cuddly to hold on to in the weeks that lay ahead. Little Squiffles became a symbol of hope and comfort, a constant reminder of God's love for me.

In Psalm 139, David marvels at how intimately God knows each one of us. "You know all my actions," he exclaims. "Even before I speak, you already know what I will say" (vv. 3–4 GNT). He goes on to point out that there is no way we can hide from God. "I could ask the darkness to hide me or the light around me to turn into night, but even darkness is not dark for you" (vv. 11–12).

When life gets tough, how wonderful to know we have a God who never loses sight of us. He will not disown us if we behave badly, nor will he ignore us when we panic. He knows each of us more completely than we know ourselves. He knows just what we need to cope in all situations, including cancer.

- Do you have a soft toy or pet to cuddle when the lights go out? If not, whom can you ask to get you one?
- God knows what you need before you ask. How does that make you feel?
- When did God provide an answer before you recognized the need?

Some months after my treatment, I learned of many situations where people who have survived trauma receive solace from a gift such as Stephen's. Deep inside each hurting person is a frightened child who needs the comfort and love that a cuddly toy can offer. That included me. And I suspect it includes you.

**LET'S PRAY:** Loving Father, you know me so well. Thank you that you understand my needs. Help me not to be too proud to accept offers of help and comfort. Amen.

*Your Father knows what you need before you ask him.*

MATTHEW 6:8

# 19

# A Long Wait

**READ:** *John 5:1-9*

The day after breast surgery, Beulah, a visitor from Reach for Recovery, came to see me. She introduced herself, then said cheerfully, "Give us a year of your life, and we will give you your life back."

I didn't want to give anyone a year of my life. I was far too busy. I begrudged the time I spent in the hospital and longed to be back in my crazy, overcommitted world. When I thought of what lay ahead, tentacles of fear coiled around my insides. I pushed those thoughts down and prayed for the Lord to help me. God knew I couldn't possibly wait twelve months to be well.

Then I read of a man who waited thirty-eight years.

The Pool of Bethesda was near the Sheep Gate leading into the walled city of Jerusalem. According to common belief, an angel periodically disturbed the water. The first person into the water after the angel's visit received healing.

Many crippled and diseased people lay in the shadows of the five stone colonnades that surrounded the pool. One of them had been crippled since his birth thirty-eight long years ago. What prompted Jesus to stop and heal that man when there were so many others in need of healing?

I'm impressed that the man showed patience and replied to Jesus with respect. He didn't demand or even plead. He stated his situation simply, perhaps with a tone of resignation.

It seems likely that he didn't hold out much hope of ever receiving healing. Yet something about Jesus's command to "rise, take up your bed and walk" seemed to resonate in him. He didn't hesitate. He clambered to his feet and he walked.

Amazing! He didn't say, "I can't. I'm a cripple." He simply got up and walked.

I longed for that same sort of miracle: "Shirley, rise up, cancel your treatment, and return to work." Could the Lord do that? I knew he could. But until then, I had to have patience and wait. At least it wouldn't be for thirty-eight years.

- What would you like Jesus to say to you today?
- How would you feel if you heard his voice and knew it was him?
- If he came and stood in front of you, what would *you* say to him?

Why do some people survive cancer when others don't? I have no idea. But I believe God is sovereign, and in some difficult-to-understand way, he has a plan for each life. What's more, it's up to him to make sure I hear what he wants of me.

LET'S PRAY: Lord Jesus, I long to hear I don't have cancer—that it's all some ghastly mistake. If that's not to be, I'd love to hear you say, "Rise, and never be ill again." Nevertheless, grant me patience. Give me the courage to go through whatever you have planned for me. Amen.

*If we hope for what we do not yet have, we wait for it patiently.*

ROMANS 8:25

# 20

## Against All Odds

READ: *Judges 7:8-15*

It was frightening enough to learn I had cancer, but the bad news didn't end there. After the operation, my surgeon told me the tumor was aggressive and had started to spread. As a result of lymph node involvement, the odds were stacked against me.

God did not allow me to remain discouraged. He sent friends to support and pray for me. When I hit my lowest moments, God brought the right visitors to cheer or encourage me. All along the wall next to my hospital bed stood beautiful arrangements of flowers, and I had already received so many cards I had to store them in my bedside cabinet.

When I thought of the fearsome enemy of cancer, I often felt overwhelmed and defenseless. Yet when I felt afraid, I could look at all the flowers and cards and remember the many prayers going up for me. I didn't know the outcome, but I felt assured that the obvious odds were not an issue. I had God on my side.

I reread the story of Gideon and his 32,000 soldiers who were about to confront the mighty battalion of Midianites. Imagine the tension in this reluctant warrior's mind when God insisted they cut their numbers down to only 300.

God knew how this order discouraged Gideon, so he told him to go down to the enemy camp. Terrified, Gideon and his servant, Purah, sneaked to the edge of the camp where they overheard two men discussing a dream. It seemed the enemy soldiers not only recognized God was with the Israelites, they expected them to win the battle. How this must have encouraged Gideon and Purah.

Sure enough, Gideon's tiny army overcame the odds in the most unlikely ways. The Israelites were victorious over the powerful Midianite army. Why? They had God on their side.

- When has the Lord fought a battle with or for you?
- How do you feel about being on God's side?
- What can you stick on your mirror to remind you that God is on your side?

Sometimes the Lord allows us to go through tough times so we learn to rely upon him. If life always seemed easy, we'd be tempted to try to manage on our own, without God. We might fail to see our need of a strong and mighty deliverer.

LET'S PRAY: Almighty God, thank you that even when the odds are stacked against me, nothing is too tough for you. Please go ahead of me into the battle against cancer. Help me to be conscious of your presence throughout today. Amen.

*No, in all these things we are more than conquerors through him who loved us.*

ROMANS 8:37

# 21

# Trip to Heaven

READ: *Luke 7:31-35*

Jesus enjoyed dinner parties. He went to weddings and visited people at home. The Pharisees resented him because he had fun. They expected him to be stiff and formal like they were. But Jesus never tried to impress. He lived a normal, open life for all to see.

The first day after surgery, I dozed in bed, vaguely aware of the other patients in the eight-bed ward. They remained strangers.

After lunch, the nurse gave me an injection for pain. Visiting time was an hour away. I had to get some sleep.

"If anyone comes to see me," I said to the nurse, "please say I've died and gone to heaven." I ignored the sudden silence in the ward as I pulled the sheet over my head to shut out the light. "I'll be back in time for visiting," I added. I didn't think of the significance of a sheet over a person's face. Nor did it occur to me that others might not be familiar with the joking comment we often used in our family. I fell asleep almost immediately.

When I awoke, visitors were streaming in. No one had dared interfere with my brief sojourn in heaven.

After visiting hours, I noticed a change in the ward.

"What's wrong with your arm?" one of the patients asked as she looked at my sling.

"Oh nothing," I said cheerfully. "I have breast cancer."

The stunned silence that followed my disclosure broke as the ladies started to share their own diagnoses. From then on, we looked out for one another. At suppertime, Sheila, who was recovering from major abdominal surgery, noticed my one-handed struggle to cut my meat. She gripped her stomach as she hobbled over to help. The patients watched each others' IV drips. We gave messages to visitors. Those of us who were able to walk filled the water jugs of those who couldn't. We shared our chocolates and cookies.

My short trip to heaven accomplished more than just a rest for me. By being myself, silly sense of humor and all, I had formed bridges between us. This changed a bunch of unhappy strangers into a group of friends with a common purpose: to get well and go home.

- Why do you think God created laughter?
- Do people see the real you, or do you put on an act?
- Who do you think your visitors come to visit, you or a pretend person?

If I sense someone is putting on an act for me, I become uneasy. I want people to relax and be themselves. When we behave naturally, others relax and relationships are formed or strengthened.

**LET'S PRAY:** Lord God, sometimes it's hard to be cheerful. Help me to be real or at least to smile at the people I come in contact with. Amen.

*[There is] a time to weep and a time to laugh, a time to mourn and a time to dance.*

ECCLESIASTES 3:4

# 22

# The Clay Lamp

READ: *Matthew 5:13-16*

The Christmas before cancer, our son Stephen gave us a beautiful clay lamp painted burgundy and gold. Shaped like a giant vase, it held only one bulb. Yet its light shone through small diamond-shaped holes carved through the clay, as well as through its wide-open top. We put it on a table in the corner of our sitting room where everyone could see it.

Shortly after I returned home from the hospital, I sat in the sitting room one evening near dusk. Someone had placed a book on top of the lamp, covering the main opening. I looked at the small diamond patterns reflected on the wall and remembered how Jesus told his disciples, "Your light must shine before people" (Matt. 5:16 GNT). My mind slipped back to the period in the hospital.

During that dark time immediately after the tumor was removed, my body felt broken. The surgeon insisted that my left arm remain strapped to my chest in a sling for over a week postoperatively. I struggled to move with an intravenous drip in my right arm, my left arm in a sling, and two rubber drains coming from the left side of my chest. Yet after the first two days I could walk and help others who were still confined to bed. I didn't *try* to behave like a Christian. My normal upbeat nature shone through, and I brought light to the atmosphere in that surgical ward.

"Nothing could quench your light," I said to the Lord as I remembered those days. "The beautiful thing is, I didn't have to switch it on. It was just there."

I felt encouraged by this thought. I just had to be me. I had the light of Jesus inside of me, and it automatically shone out to the people near me. Even if the anesthetic, drugs, or pain dimmed my main light for a short period, like the book on top of that lamp, God's light still shone out through the cracks.

- In what way does God's light shine through you?
- What prevents Christ's light from shining out of you to others?
- Who are the ones closest to you who need to see that light?

Nothing takes God by surprise, not even cancer. As we heal from surgery, we can do little to repair the brokenness, but we can allow him to shine through the cracks. Then others will see his light and receive blessing. You don't have to *try* to help them; you just need to allow Christ to shine through you.

**LET'S PRAY:** Lord God, you saw this tumor develop from the first errant cell. You have allowed these cracks to appear in my body. Please shine through them to the people around me. Amen.

*We have this treasure in jars of clay to show that this all-surpassing power is from God and not from us.*

2 CORINTHIANS 4:7

# 23

# All One Body

**READ:** *1 Corinthians 12:12-26*

Shortly after coming home from the hospital, I had a visit from my friend Barbara. Devastated by the news of my cancer, she was amazed to find me lighthearted as I related funny stories from the ward.

Suddenly she stood and said, "I must go. I don't want to exhaust you. Before I leave, may I pray with you?"

"Yes, of course," I replied. "Thank you."

She came across the room and knelt close to my chair. She took my hands and started to pray. Tears ran down her cheeks, dripping onto our hands. Eventually she was unable to pray further. She sank her head onto our clasped hands and sobbed. When she showed no sign of being able to continue her prayer, I extricated one soggy hand from under the pile and placed it on her hair.

"Father, I ask you to bring comfort and strength to Barbara as she struggles to cope with my diagnosis," I prayed. "Help her to trust you with my life."

How incredible. My friend loved me so much that *she* needed prayer. She came to visit with the intent of supporting me, yet I ended up helping her. Barbara's visit left me feeling loved and more aware of others.

The Corinthian church was full of problems. People who should have worked together were disagreeing and wanting to do their own thing. That's why Paul wrote 1 Corinthians. It's his letter to the congregation in which he points out how the members should behave within the church. He tells them they belong to one body and paints the ridiculous scenario of an ear that refuses to be part of the body because it's not an eye. "If our bodies were only an eye," he says, "we couldn't hear a thing. And if they were only an ear, we couldn't smell a thing" (1 Cor. 12:17 CEV).

Paul points out that just as it takes many parts to make one body, it takes many parts, or people, to make a congregation. In the same way that body parts must work together for a person to be healthy, so the people within a congregation must work together for a church to be healthy. We are all different—but we need one another.

- In what ways can you reach out to your loved ones to help them deal with your diagnosis?
- When friends come to visit, many of them are hurting. How can you encourage them?
- Is there someone you can pray for who is affected by your cancer?

Physically we can't escape the effects of cancer or of the treatment. Emotionally we are shattered. Those who love us are also devastated, but they don't have the prayer support we have. Look for ways to encourage them, and in the process you yourself will be uplifted.

**LET'S PRAY:** Father, thank you for friends and loved ones. Help me to be aware of their needs, and show me where they need my support and encouragement. Amen.

*If one part [of the body] suffers, every part suffers with it.*

1 CORINTHIANS 12:26

# 24

# Friends in Deed

READ: *Acts 9:26-31*

When I first returned home, I had a never-ending stream of visitors. I appreciated each person and chattered incessantly with everyone. I'm sure people often left confused by my cheerfulness and apparent lack of concern about my cancer.

They couldn't have been more wrong. For some reason, I often felt ostracized and desperately wanted to be normal. I didn't want pity, but neither did I want people to pretend there was nothing wrong.

Some people didn't know what to say, so they simply said nothing and gave the impression they weren't interested. Others cross-examined me, prying for details I hadn't yet processed for myself. Members of the medical profession, who in the past always offered a pill to make an illness go away, were hesitant, contradictory, and indirect with their answers. If ever I needed a true friend, it was then.

Several people stepped forward. Sheila watered and tended my plants; Margie lent me two blouses that opened down the front; George collected medicine from across town; Bert found a rubber stress ball for my arm exercises; Theresa took my son to the dentist when he developed an abscess; Noelene washed and groomed my tangled Maltese poodle; and many others cooked and delivered hot meals. And so the list went on. These people moved beyond the status of visitor and showed themselves to be friends in deed.

In the New Testament, Saul needed a friend. Once this bully had viciously pursued and persecuted Christians, but he had been out of the public eye for three years. Now he had returned and claimed to be a believer. It's likely that many people suspected him of being a spy. Others despised him for his past actions. When he committed his life to Jesus, Saul had turned against the Jewish leaders he had previously supported. He joined the opposition, and his former colleagues regarded him as a traitor.

Distrusted by his fellow believers and under threat from his former co-workers, Saul needed a friend. Then Barnabas, whose name means "son of comfort," stepped forward. A well-liked and respected member of the community, he came alongside Saul and persuaded the apostles to accept him. The reassured disciples welcomed the newcomer into their group. Saul, who was renamed Paul, could have refused Barnabas's help, but he recognized his need of a true friend. The two men became close and often worked together.

- Which friends have shown you love in practical ways?
- Are you sending out mixed signals? Do people understand your true needs?
- Whom can you speak to about your disease and treatment? Whom can you ask for help?

Some people will come alongside without any prompting; others may need your assistance. Share some information or ask them for help. One of your visitors may want to be your friend but doesn't know how.

**LET'S PRAY:** Loving Father, thank you for friends. Help me to allow people to draw close to me at this time. Show me how to be a friend. Amen.

*A friend loves at all times, and a brother is born for a time of adversity.*

PROVERBS 17:17

Turn to appendix 3 on page 205 for a list of suggestions you can share with your friends. Let's help them to help us.

# 25

# Get Back on the Beam

**READ:** *John 21:15-19*

Soon after I returned home, I watched an episode of *Touched by an Angel*, one of my favorite TV programs. The story centered on a family hit by cancer. Panic built up inside me. I wanted to scream at Rob, "Switch it off!" Embarrassed by my weakness, I remained quiet. Rob later admitted he had the same thoughts. A lack of communication—and the show ran its course.

In the story, the family struggled to come to terms with the loss of their husband and father. The man left behind a young teenage daughter, a gifted gymnast. He had never missed one of her meets, and now the girl faced a major competition without her dad's support. She did well in each event. For the final test, she ran into the arena and vaulted onto the beam. She performed a brilliant routine. Then it happened. As she landed on the beam after a high somersault, her foot slipped. She crashed to the sawdust and lay there sobbing.

Monica, one of the angels in the series, appeared next to her. "Get up!" she urged. "You've got to get back on the beam." The girl lay still for a while, then slowly rose to her feet. With tears streaming down her face, she leaped back onto the beam and steadied herself.

She completed her routine with a flawless performance that was followed by tumultuous applause from the excited audience.

When the show finished, I felt emotionally sick.

"Why didn't we switch it off?" I demanded of Rob. Reluctantly I recognized that the Lord had wanted us to watch this episode.

"So what's the Lord saying? That I'm going to die of cancer? And you guys must go on without me?"

"No," Rob replied. "I believe God is saying, 'You've got to get back on the beam!'"

"I'm not aware I've fallen off the beam," I retorted.

"Maybe not yet. But perhaps the Lord is preparing us for when you do."

I had no intention of falling off any beam. We had a time of prayer and went to bed.

A few days later, I had a horrible day. Everything frustrated me and I crumbled. Rob held me while I sobbed, then spoke gently. "Enough, Shirl. Dry your tears. It's time to get back on the beam."

- Where do you struggle the most in your cancer journey?
- What is your biggest fear?
- Have you fallen off the beam? If so, how will you get back on?

Sometimes we need loved ones or friends who will say, "Enough. Stop crying and move forward." It's okay to succumb to grief. It's normal to feel afraid. There's a time to cry, but then there's a time to get back on the beam.

LET'S PRAY: Father, sometimes it all seems too much for me. When things get me down, help me to hold tight to your hand, pick myself up, and get back on the beam. Amen.

*He heals the brokenhearted and binds up their wounds.*

PSALM 147:3

# 26

## It's Too Much!

READ: *Matthew 14:25-32*

I handled my immediate postoperative situation well. Sure, at times I felt tossed around and buffeted by winds of panic. But I didn't rant and rave, nor did I cry. Visitors marveled at my calm assurance of God's control.

One morning I awoke uptight. The wound on my arm and chest throbbed and the sling that bound my arm to my body irritated me. I walked past my younger son's bedroom and glanced in. He hadn't opened his curtains before leaving for college.

Annoyed, I shoved at his door with my good arm and stormed into the room. The door boomeranged off a tower of books piled precariously on his bookcase and slammed into my damaged arm. The protruding door handle punched me on the breast at the exact point of my incision. Books tumbled to the floor.

"Ow!" I wailed. I threw myself onto the bed and sobbed, cradling my bandaged arm to my chest.

Rob flew into the room. "What on earth's wrong?" he asked in alarm. He held me close while I cried and cried. The pent-up tears of the past two weeks soaked into his shirt.

Peter would have understood. After a long, tiring day, Jesus sent his disciples across the Sea of Galilee while he climbed a nearby hill to spend time in prayer. In the early hours of the morning, a sudden storm sprang up. Waves driven by a fierce wind tossed their little boat up and down. The experienced fishermen were petrified.

When Jesus appeared out of the spray walking on the water, they screamed in terror. I don't blame them.

"Don't worry!" Jesus called. "It's me, Jesus."

Impetuous Peter shouted back, "Lord, if it's really you, tell me to come to you."

Jesus responded, "Come on then."

Without further thought, Peter clambered over the edge of the boat and walked confidently to Jesus. The waves churned around his feet. Suddenly he realized the strength of the wind. He called out in fear as he started to sink. Of course, we know what happened. Jesus shot out his arm and caught Peter, then helped him back into the boat. Yet even that is amazing. Jesus, who was standing on the turbulent water, caught a panicking Peter and rescued him. Surely nothing is too difficult for the Lord.

- What one thing terrifies you the most about cancer?
- Would you rather try to walk to Jesus and have him rescue you, or stay in the boat?
- Why?

This was the first time I allowed my emotions to have the upper hand, but it certainly wouldn't be the last. We need to cry out to the Lord when we feel the waves of terror or anger crashing around us. He is always within reach, ready to stretch out his hand to steady us. Nothing is too difficult for him.

**LET'S PRAY:** Lord God, sometimes I watch the size of the waves instead of watching you. Help me to keep my hand in yours as I try to stay afloat in this stormy time. Thank you. Amen.

*I am the LORD, the God of all mankind. Is anything too hard for me?*

JEREMIAH 32:27

# 27

# Long Toenails and All

READ: *Luke 19:28-40*

Within days of my surgery, I needed to cut my toenails. With my arm strapped to my body, I couldn't even reach my toes let alone cut the nails. My friend Brenda came to visit and offered to help. She sat next to me on the settee and held my feet in her hands. She laughed when she discovered how ticklish I am. Then she cut my nails for me. When she finished, she led me to the bathroom where she washed my hair.

I found it difficult to allow her to do these things for me. Yet it's not only important for us to allow others to show love in practical ways, it's also important for them. According to the Scriptures, when others do something for us, it's as if they're doing it for the Lord.

When Jesus entered Jerusalem, he sent his disciples to fetch a young colt that had never been ridden. As the creature stomped its feet in the dust, the disciples threw their cloaks onto its back. How could Jesus get onto this excited beast? He couldn't do it alone. He needed their help.

Their strong arms gripped him and, perhaps on the count of three, they heaved him onto the animal's back. He could have tried to get on by himself, but he allowed his friends to come close. He let them hold him, lift him, and steady him.

During the next days, there were many such times. The disciples were there when he broke the bread and poured the wine. They allowed Jesus to wash their feet. They saw him cry. At least one of the disciples, and a number of his followers, stood nearby in silent support when he died. Some would help to lower his broken body from the cross and lay it in a tomb.

- Why is it so difficult to let others help you in intimate ways?
- Can you think of a time when you allowed, or refused to allow, someone to draw close to you?
- Is there an area where you need help right now? Whom will you ask for help?

Cancer is a leveler of persons. Our independence is temporarily destroyed, and we need to lean on others for support. Allowing people to draw close and do tasks that we would normally do for ourselves is difficult. We would much rather be doing things for others. As hard as it may be, we must let people see the real us—long toenails and all.

**LET'S PRAY:** Loving Father, thank you for showing me by your own example that I need to allow others to draw close. Please bring people into my life whom I can trust, who will help me when I need them. Bless them for their love and care. Amen.

*If one of you says to them, "Go in peace; keep warm and well fed," but does nothing about their physical needs, what good is it? In the same way, faith by itself, if it is not accompanied by action, is dead.*

JAMES 2:16–17

# 28

# A Work of Art

READ: *Acts 18:1-3*

I loved to do crafts. I used to make greeting cards as a hobby and send them to friends and even to people I had never met. When the news got out about my diagnosis, I received a flood of cards, many of them homemade. My most treasured card came all the way from the jungles of Venezuela and was made by Debbie, my daughter. She assured me that my son-in-law and two precious grandchildren sent their love. They were all concerned, they missed us, and they were praying. I stood that card on my bedside table where I could see it whenever I lay down.

I appreciated every card, but there were not enough available surfaces to display so many. So a few days after my return home, I asked my husband to buy a roll of brown paper and a tube of glue. Clumsily, I knelt down on the floor and spread the brown paper on the carpet. With one arm still in a sling, it took me most of the morning to stick all the cards onto the paper.

My arms ached and my back hurt as I wriggled around the carpet, trying to confine the glue to the paper. After I stuck the last card in place, I gazed at it with pride. Rob and our youngest son, David, mounted the montage on the wall for me. Each time I looked at it I felt a sense of accomplishment, and I felt loved.

As a work of art it wasn't much, but I had done it myself. The act of being creative encouraged me. I realized how important it was for me to stay active. I knew it would be a while until I could return to my work as a nurse, but I determined to use my time in constructive ways.

Paul was another person who didn't like to waste time. He was not only a well-educated teacher and a theologian, he also knew how to work with his hands. One day he left Athens and went to Corinth. There he met a Jew from Italy by the name of Aquila and his wife, Priscilla. They became firm friends and discovered they shared a common interest: they were all tentmakers by trade. Their craft became a means of reaching out to others as well as giving them a sense of accomplishment.

- How do you use your free time? Are you creative?
- What hobby are you able to work on that you can pick up and put down again without hassle?
- Is there a new craft you can learn?

If you have to be away from work for an extended recovery time, maybe now is a good time to learn something new. Take an interest in a fresh subject. Do some research on different hobbies. The Lord has made us to be creative, and the sense of achievement will help to lift your spirits.

**LET'S PRAY:** Lord God, you are the great Creator and you made me in your image. Show me something I can tackle that will give me a sense of accomplishment. Thank you for my gifts and talents. Help me to find ways to use them, even when I don't feel like it. Amen.

*May the God of hope fill you with all joy and peace as you trust in him, so that you may overflow with hope by the power of the Holy Spirit.*

ROMANS 15:13

# 29

# Unworthy, but Loved

**READ:** *Matthew 9:10-13*

As a pastor's wife, I was surrounded by praying people. Across the world, prayer groups asked the Lord to heal me. I tried to pray with faith myself, yet deep down I had no conviction that healing would be the outcome. I didn't deserve it.

Slowly I came to realize that if the Lord only healed those who deserved to be healed, no one would qualify. It was God's decision whether he would heal me here on earth or whether he would take me home to heaven. Either way, I would soon be well again—not because I deserved to be, but because Jesus came to earth for people like me.

During Jesus's earthly ministry, many disreputable characters gathered around him. One evening he and his followers were eating supper in the home of Matthew, who was a tax collector. The Pharisees asked the disciples, "What kind of example is this from your Teacher, acting cozy with crooks and riff-raff?" (Matt. 9:11 Message). They didn't speak to Jesus himself but talked behind his back. Yet Jesus overheard and shot back his own question: "Who needs a doctor: the healthy or the sick?" (9:12).

The Savior didn't come to heal those who were well. He didn't come to show people the way to heaven if they thought they had it all figured out and refused his help. He didn't plan to reach those who thought they deserved his touch; his plan was to reach the undeserving. In other words, he came for those with real needs. That means he came for me.

- Can you think of reasons why you're not good enough to receive healing?
- If you handed a list of your reasons to Jesus, what do you think he'd say?
- What would you like to do with your life after cancer?

The Lord chose to give me back my life, not because I deserved it, but because he had work for me to do. As a Christian, I know that one day I will still experience physical death and I will go to live in heaven. It's a win-win situation. Whether I had gone to be with the Lord the year of my cancer treatment or whether I remain on earth for many more years, I don't deserve either. Jesus came to bring us salvation and healing because he loves us, not because we deserve it.

**LET'S PRAY:** Lord God, thank you for loving me so much. Help me to remember that I don't need to earn my healing or my salvation. Thank you that one day I'll be safe in heaven with you. Help me to rejoice and not be afraid. Amen.

*But seek first his kingdom and his righteousness, and all these things will be given to you as well.*

MATTHEW 6:33

# 30

## Overcoming Challenges

READ: *Luke 5:17-24*

Immediately after surgery, my left arm was encased in a navy sling with straps that held it tight against my body. When the physiotherapist saw the sling, she complained.

"That surgeon of yours again," she muttered. "He always does this, and then the patient battles to move her arm afterward." Right at that moment, I wasn't worried. Movement was agony, and I was happy to have the sling.

Eight days later, I had to take the sling off and start to exercise my arm in preparation for radiation. That's when the fun began. I could barely move my arm, nor could I straighten my elbow.

"You have to be able to stretch your arm until your fingers reach the ear on the opposite side," the physiotherapist instructed. "Stand close to the door, then walk your fingers up the surface." She had to be joking. I could barely *reach* the door.

Back home, I prayed for guidance. Then I had an idea of another way to do the exercises. Every few hours throughout the day and whenever I woke at night, I worked on my muscles, using my strong arm to help my weaker one. I relaxed my left arm and gripped my left wrist with my right hand. Slowly I pulled my arm into a new position. That stretched the hurting muscles and tendons without making them do extra work. It was painful but doable. Slowly the movement returned. The following week the oncologist cleared me for radiation. It wasn't easy, but creativity helped me through the crisis.

One day when Jesus was preaching in Peter's home, some men showed great creativity. They brought their crippled friend on a stretcher in hopes that the miracle worker would heal him. When they arrived, they couldn't get near Jesus because of the crowd. The resourceful friends made their way up the outside staircase to the flat roof. Houses in those days were often built around a courtyard. A detachable roof covered the area during the winter and could be removed in the summer. The friends knelt down and removed the tiles. Opening the roof above the speaker's head, they lowered the stretcher to the room below.

Jesus was delighted to see the faith not only of the crippled man but of his creative friends. How thrilled the men on the roof must have been as they watched their friend rise to his feet, pick up his stretcher, and walk out of the house a well man.

- In what ways does the story of the paralyzed man encourage you?
- Which instruction from your medical team do you find difficult to follow?
- Is there a creative way around the problem? Give it some thought now.

When we are tempted to say "I can't do this!" we need to remember the crippled man's friends. They didn't give up and neither should we. Perhaps the "normal" way of doing things is not working. Then be creative. If it's important enough, you will find a way. Ask the Lord to show you.

**LET'S PRAY:** Lord God, sometimes it's easier to give up. Help me with the problem I face today, and show me a creative way to overcome any obstacle. Thank you. Amen.

*I can do all this through him who gives me strength.*

PHILIPPIANS 4:13

# 31

## Tattoos Are Forever

READ: *John 20:24-29*

No one warned me in advance that I would receive four permanent tattoos on my chest prior to radiation. Each one is only the size of a small pinhead, but they are there forever. When I wear a bathing suit, two of the marks are easily visible. I can never forget I had radiation.

Isn't that how we should be as Christians? When people look at us, they should be able to immediately recognize that we belong to Jesus. Cancer treatment is exhausting, unpleasant, and causes horrible side effects. I prayed constantly that I would continue to be a good witness to the people I came into contact with. It wasn't always easy.

Jesus also received permanent marks that will always remind him of what he went through at Calvary.

Thomas, one of the twelve disciples, wasn't present when the risen Lord appeared to the others in the upper room. He announced that unless he saw for himself the nail prints in Jesus's hands, he wouldn't believe his companions had seen him. A week later the Lord again appeared to the disciples. He went straight to Thomas and showed him his hands. Thomas knelt in worship, proclaiming, "My Lord and my God!" Although Jesus was alive, his hands still held the marks of crucifixion.

- Did you receive tattoos as part of your radiation therapy? How do you feel about them?

- If Thomas told *you* he wouldn't believe Jesus had risen unless he saw the nail prints for himself, what would you say?
- When people talk to you, what shows them you belong to Jesus Christ?

We can look at our tattoos from cancer treatment as awful reminders of a ghastly time in our lives, or we can use them as reminders of what God brought us through. I choose the latter. How about you?

**LET'S PRAY:** Lord God, thank you that you bear the scars on your hands as an eternal proof of what you went through at Calvary. Help me to always view my cancer and treatment scars as proof of what you did in my life during this difficult time. Amen.

*On my own body are scars that prove I belong to Christ Jesus.*

GALATIANS 6:17 CEV

# 32

## I Feel like a Grasshopper

READ: *Numbers 13:26-33*

For forty days the Israelite spies surveyed Canaan. They got to know its terrain, its towns, and its people. Before them lay a wonderful land, but the inhabitants were "giants" and the spies saw themselves as mere "grasshoppers." Of the twelve men who entered the land, only Joshua and Caleb believed that with God on their side, the army of Israel could conquer Canaan. "We can certainly do it!" Caleb urged the nation.

Sadly, Israel listened to the other ten men who had their eyes on the giants. It cost them forty years of wandering in the wilderness. Of the adults who made up the original group, only Joshua and Caleb would eventually enter Canaan.

When I faced the giants of cancer, out-of-control cell counts, and emotional roller coasters, I felt insignificant and defenseless. When I entered the room that housed the giant radiation machines, I felt overwhelmed. Each time I received a dose of chemotherapy I was reminded of my fragility and my mortality.

I learned how important it is to focus on God. When I looked at the machines, the intravenous drips, and the other challenges I faced, I lost courage. I knew I couldn't win—and I was right. But when I looked at God, the giants didn't seem so big after all. I knew that in his strength I could certainly do it.

- What giants have you already overcome in your cancer battle?
- What specific giant are you facing at the moment?

- How does that giant look when you compare it to God?

I wish I could say I lost my fear of giants, but I didn't. They continued to appear along the way, and I often found myself reverting to grasshopper mode. Yet when I remembered to compare the giants with an almighty God, I found the courage to once again move forward. In God's strength I could battle the giants. Alone, I was just a grasshopper.

**LET'S PRAY:** Lord, I'm sorry for the times I try to do things on my own and then wonder why I'm so afraid. Help me to remember my dependence on you. Grant me the courage I need to face the giants of cancer. Amen.

*Not that we are competent in ourselves to claim anything for ourselves, but our competence comes from God.*

2 CORINTHIANS 3:5

# 33

# A Strange Place to Worship

READ: *Acts 16:16–34*

Paul and Silas had been arrested in the city of Philippi. After being severely flogged, they were thrown into the innermost cell of the prison. Their feet were placed in stocks. Yet in the middle of the night they kept the other prisoners awake as they prayed and sang praises to God. A prison cell—what a strange place to worship.

On the day of my first radiation treatment I was terrified. The therapists helped me into position on a steel bed and instructed me to hold a handle above my head. They clanged the door shut and left me alone.

As I stared at the blank ceiling, I remembered a dentist we visited when our children were young. He had a cartoon painted on the ceiling above the chair. You only saw it when the chair tipped back. How I wished for a cartoon on this ceiling.

"Oh Lord, help," I muttered. "I'm scared."

"Look to me," I sensed his reply. "You've taught others to praise me in all circumstances. Now do it yourself."

Praise him? Now?

Frantic, I gripped the handle and held my breath. How could I praise him? I remembered a song about praising God no matter where I was. The machines started to hum. Petrified, I began to sing in a wavery voice. The words spoke of Christ's love surrounding me like a sea. I squeezed my eyes shut. I imagined the bed where I lay to be a tiny island. I visualized seawater lapping against the legs of the bed.

My arm hurt and my body ached from the awkward position, yet I forced myself to concentrate on the words. I imagined Jesus smiling down on me from the blank ceiling, accepting my praise. Over the next six weeks this became my routine. Every day I spent several minutes on my back staring into the face of Jesus on the once-blank ceiling. Every day I tried to think of a different song. Every day I ended up singing the same one. I often thought the Lord must be getting awfully sick of that short song, but since he didn't prompt me with another, I just kept on singing. My mind joined in the game, and I often thought I heard water lapping around me as I lay perched on the platform, surrounded by the love of Jesus. While my body was barraged with destructive rays, my mind and emotions were lifted high by my Savior.

- You can dwell on the unpleasant parts of treatment or on Jesus and his love. Which makes you feel better?
- What song of praise can you sing to Jesus today?
- Where do you need to see Jesus the most? Imagine him there.

Scripture assures us that the Lord knows where we are at all times. He knows exactly what we're going through. He also knows that the best way to get our minds off the tough things is to get our eyes on him. What better way is there than to praise him?

**LET'S PRAY:** Lord Jesus, I thank you for bringing me this far. I rejoice that you are here with me. Show me how to praise and worship you wherever I am, even in strange places. Amen.

*Worship the LORD in the splendor of his holiness.*

1 CHRONICLES 16:29

# 34

# Bring in the Artillery

**READ:** *1 Samuel 17:38-50*

It had been several weeks since my surgery. The tumor was gone; however, because my lymph nodes were involved, I faced radiation and then two courses of chemotherapy.

The afternoon following my first session of radiation, I rested on my bed and thought about the time I had spent under the huge machines. It occurred to me that my fight against cancer was like a war.

The first wave of the war was like hand-to-hand combat, when the infantry came in and destroyed Goliath, my nickname for the initial tumor. Now we had brought in tanks, machine guns, and heavy artillery—in the form of powerful radiation machines.

The giant that had served under my enemy, Satan, was now dead. However, there was a strong likelihood of further rogue cells in my body. I saw these leftover cancer cells as enemy soldiers that had survived the first front of the war. They needed to be routed from wherever they were hiding. The rays fired from the massive machines would clear the local area of the enemy.

If this all sounds highly imaginative, that is exactly my point. I started to use my imagination to promote healing instead of death. As I lay under the machines, I mentally directed the rays to the hiding cancer cells. I cheered them on as I sang. The more positive thoughts I cultivated, the more confident I became. The more time I spent encouraging the machines in their work, the less time I had left for negative emotions.

In the well-known story of David and Goliath, we read of how the Philistine giant taunted the young shepherd boy. Yet it only took one smooth stone in the hands of a slingshot expert and guided by God, and the giant lay dead. That was one small victory for the Israelites, but the war still needed to be won. The rest of the Philistine army had to be dealt with. So too, the removal of my tumor was a victory for me, but it wasn't enough. The rest of the enemy still had to be eliminated.

- In what ways do the radiation machines compare with weapons of warfare?
- How can you use *your* mind in your fight against cancer?
- During what times are you inclined to be negative? What praise song can you use during such times?

I once read an acrostic for the word *fear*: false evidence appearing real. I determined to take up the shield of faith against all false evidence and negative thoughts and instead fill my mind with positive, victorious concepts.

LET'S PRAY: Lord God, I call you Lord because you're in command of my life. Help me to remember that as my Commander in Chief I can trust you with my body and my future. Amen.

*The one who is in you is greater than the one who is in the world.*

1 JOHN 4:4

# 35

## Time Out

READ: *Mark 1:32-35*

In my pre-cancer days I never took afternoon naps. I was too busy. However, during radiation treatment I found that by midday I couldn't keep going. After lunch I headed for the bedroom, lay down, and picked up a book. Often I fell asleep.

Candy, our fluffy Maltese poodle, and Yoda, our ginger tomcat, soon learned the new routine. They seemed to sense my need for undemanding company and unquestioning devotion, and they were only too happy to oblige. We had never allowed our animals on the bed, but this seemed a good time to bend the rules.

One afternoon I said to Rob, "Watch this."

I started to walk toward the bedroom. Our sleeping poodle immediately leapt to her feet. She shot past me and raced down the corridor. By the time I reached my bedroom, she stood on the bed, her tail wagging and her little pink tongue hanging out with excitement. I clambered onto the bed, and she curled up on my right side.

Before I had time to pick up my book, a languid meow came from the door. In strolled Yoda, tail erect. He jumped onto the mattress and stalked to my other side. He stretched himself out, pressing against me. I felt loved and cherished, even if somewhat cramped.

Initially I struggled with the need to rest every day. It seemed such a waste of time. Yet I came to accept that my body needed that time-out—and so did my mind. The days when I pushed through and didn't have my nap, I was out of sorts by evening and battled just to cope.

I noticed the Bible's emphasis on rest. God himself rested for an entire day after creating the world. We often read of Jesus going off on his own for a time of quiet and prayer, especially after a period of intense ministry. I struggled to teach myself to relax and accept that, at least during this period of my life, I needed time to rest and recuperate. I started to look forward to the time on my bed—and so did my pets.

- What time of day do you most need time-out?
- How can you best prepare for your break? How can you make it a priority?
- What pet or fluffy toy would love to share that time with you?

When your energy is depleted, allow yourself the luxury of relaxation. Accept this as part of the healing process and enjoy it. You and all those around you will benefit from this time—even your pets.

**LET'S PRAY:** Lord, set the pace for my day. Help me to know when to make an effort and when to take time to relax. Thank you for setting me an example of time-out. Amen.

*Come to me, all you who are weary and burdened, and I will give you rest.*

MATTHEW 11:28

# 36

## I Feel So Alone

READ: *Psalm 18:1-6*

Every day seemed to bring a new crisis. Even when I awoke eager to get up and enjoy the day, there was invariably a problem lurking in the shadows. I often felt overwhelmed and would cry out to God. Although my husband and sons were supportive, they couldn't be there for me every minute of the day. Even if they were with me, they couldn't always understand the feelings of terror or confusion that would sweep over me.

"Lord, I feel so alone!" I often cried out. Sometimes I battled with these emotions for a while before taking steps to bring them under control. I found the quickest way to pull out of these times was to put on a CD of praise music or to sit quietly and read Scripture. Often a sense of peace and assurance would well up inside me, and I would know that I wasn't alone.

God, who knows me by name, was right next to me. He had promised to walk through the waters of cancer with me. He would ensure that the flames of radiation wouldn't consume me. He wouldn't allow the rivers of chemotherapy to overwhelm me. How grateful I was that I had the assurance of his company. I wondered how people who didn't have faith in the one true God ever coped with cancer treatment.

- How does it feel knowing that God is next to you wherever you go, no matter what you face?

- What steps can you take to remind yourself of God's never-failing love for you?
- God knows you by name. What does this mean to you?

The cancer journey is a lonely one. No matter how caring your family or friends may be, there are many times of isolation when they cannot be with you. No one can climb into your thoughts and keep you company in the deepest parts of your being—no one except for Jesus. Surround yourself with gospel music, easy-to-read Christian books, anything that will help you to be constantly aware of his company.

**LET'S PRAY:** Lord, thank you so much for your amazing love. I struggle to believe that you care so much for me. Help me to grasp this as a reality, because I know what a difference it will make in how I deal with today. Amen.

*I have summoned you by name; you are mine. When you pass through the waters, I will be with you.*

ISAIAH 43:1–2

# 37

## Company in the Storm

READ: *Mark 4:35-41*

The small fishing boat tossed and groaned at the intensity of the storm. On board, experienced fishermen rowed and bailed as if their lives depended upon their efforts—which indeed they did.

Although cyclonic squalls of that nature were common on the Sea of Galilee, this one appeared to catch the men by surprise. In the stern, Jesus the landlubber slept peacefully. Didn't he understand the danger? In terror, they shook him awake.

"Don't you realize we're going to drown?" they screamed.

Jesus calmed the waves and the wind. Then he scolded the men for their lack of faith. They had obviously forgotten that he created the waves and the wind. He had no reason to be afraid. Nor did they as long as they were with him.

Many times during my year of treatment I asked the Lord to take away some unpleasant side effect. Sometimes he did. More often he calmed my fears and reminded me that he was with me. Even when he didn't remove the symptoms, he brought me peace. I sensed his presence as he kept me company through the difficult periods. Sometimes I felt terrified, but Jesus never did. He created me, and he remained in control of my circumstances, no matter the size of the waves.

- What storm is breaking about you right now? Talk to Jesus about it.

- When you see the waves approaching, what is the first thing you should do?
- Do you know someone who is afraid of the same storm? Can you offer them some encouragement?

**LET'S PRAY:** Lord Jesus, thank you that when I face a storm in my life, you are there with me, and you are never afraid. Help me to trust in you no matter how frightening the situation. Amen.

*Trust in the LORD forever, for the LORD, the LORD himself, is the Rock eternal.*

ISAIAH 26:4

# 38

## I Hate Roller Coasters!

READ: *1 Kings 19:3-13*

Elijah had never been to a fairground, but he knew all about roller coasters.

With great faith he confronted the wicked King Ahab and experienced some amazing miracles. Then his faith plunged as he turned and fled in fear for his life after threats from Queen Jezebel. What a letdown.

The great man of God became depressed to the point of wanting to die—and he slept for several days. He woke in amazement as an angel brought him food and encouraged him. He then set out for a long journey on foot, desperate to hear from God.

A sudden wind, an earthquake, and a furious fire all failed to reveal God. Then, in a period of calm, Elijah heard what he'd longed for, a word from the Lord God.

Up and down. Down and up. From heights of faith to depths of despair and back.

I could relate to Elijah.

Sometimes my emotions soared with joy only to plummet hours later as my mind filled with dread. One minute I hit a pinnacle of faith, the next I experienced a wave of panic. I would awaken with confidence that God and I together would lick this dreadful disease and I would live for many years. Then I would go into the bathroom and catch sight of my reflection in the mirror and my confidence would give way to doubt.

I soon learned that there were two good things about the so-called cancer roller coaster. First, since these mood swings were a well-documented occurrence in cancer patients, I could rest assured that my up-and-down emotions were normal and not a symptom that the cancer had spread to my brain. Second, like all true roller coasters, when I hit the bottom I could remind myself that I would shortly be on the way back up. The problem was, I never did enjoy roller coaster rides.

- How does it help to know that an emotional roller coaster is normal during cancer treatment?
- What do you like—or dislike—about roller coasters at an amusement park?
- What are some similarities you see between a roller coaster and the emotional ride you are now on?

In cancer recovery, the old adage "what goes up must come down" is also true in reverse: what goes down must come up. That applies to emotions and to blood counts. (And no, it shouldn't apply to food! If this is a problem, speak to your doctor.) Enjoy the peaks and learn to ride out the valleys in the confidence that better times are ahead.

**LET'S PRAY:** Lord God, I hate that I'm so emotionally unstable. Please help me to ride this roller coaster with dignity and calm. Remind me that you are in charge of the machinery. Amen.

*Be still, and know that I am God.*

PSALM 46:10

# 39

## Need to Focus

READ: *John 8:25-29*

I've put in for two weeks' sick leave," I had told one of my colleagues at work. "By then I should be over the surgery. If I feel well enough before then, I'll be back sooner."

We were short-staffed, and I didn't intend to be away longer than absolutely necessary. I knew that if the surgeon had to remove the entire breast it would probably take me longer to recover, but I was only thinking one day at a time. I resolved to do what the doctors required but to keep living my life to the full.

I soon discovered this didn't work. Cancer took over my life—every minute of it. With extreme tiredness came the need for more rest. Food preparation took longer. When my immunity became impaired, I couldn't just munch on an apple. I had to peel it and sometimes even cook it. Extra visitors were wonderful, but they tired me. I came to realize the wisdom of Beulah, my friend from Reach for Recovery: I needed to dedicate the time of treatment to getting well. I had to trust God with my future.

I spent more time reading the Word of God. I also read everything I could find with a positive message. When I saw a cancer-related story, the first thing I did was check the back page. If it contained a tribute to the writer who had passed on, I put the book back. I only wanted to read about people who survived.

One day as Jesus entered the town of Capernaum, a centurion came and asked him to heal his servant, who was lying paralyzed at home. Jesus healed him—from a distance. He then went into

Peter's house and found the disciple's mother-in-law extremely ill with a fever. Jesus healed her too. When evening came, we read that he cast out demons and "healed all the sick" (Matt. 8:16). The next morning Jesus and the disciples walked out of the house to discover a huge crowd of people waiting for him. There were doubtless many sick, blind, and crippled people in the crowd hoping for a touch from the Miracle Man.

When Jesus saw the crowd, he instructed the disciples to take him across the Sea of Galilee. Why did Jesus turn his back on the crowd? Surely they also needed healing.

On another occasion when the Pharisees challenged Jesus about his actions, he replied, "I do nothing on my own authority, but I say only what the Father has instructed me to say" (John 8:28 GNT). Jesus remained focused on one thing—doing what his Father told him. If his Father told him to heal, Jesus healed. If his Father told him to cross the lake, Jesus crossed the lake.

- What issues sidetrack you from your mission to get well?
- Which visitors help you feel good?
- What or who should you put on hold for the moment?

As I looked at Jesus's example, I realized it was time to put all my energy into survival. I had to focus on health not disease. Most of all, I needed to do what the Lord showed me to do and not allow myself to get involved in other issues.

**LET'S PRAY:** Lord Jesus, only you know why I'm going through this. Please help me to keep my eyes on you. Show me how to focus on the positive and not allow myself to be distracted. Amen.

*Let us keep our eyes fixed on Jesus, on whom our faith depends from beginning to end.*

HEBREWS 12:2 GNT

# 40

## Over the Edge

READ: *Psalm 3:1-8*

I once read about a man who stumbled over a cliff. As he plummeted toward the rocks below, he grabbed hold of a small tree growing out of the side of the cliff.

"Help!" he yelled as he dangled from the branch. "Help! Is there anyone up there who can help me?"

After what seemed like a long time, he heard a loud voice.

"Don't be afraid—I am here."

"Oh, thank goodness!" the man responded in relief. "Who are you?"

"I am the almighty God," boomed the response.

That sounded like good news. Surely God would be able to help him.

"Quick, what must I do?" the man screamed.

"Let go of the branch and my everlasting arms will catch you," came the reply.

After a marked pause, the man called out, "Help! Is there anyone else up there who can help me?"

I often felt the same way during my cancer journey. I frequently received confirmation of God's almighty power at work in my life. When my white cell count plummeted, I would read an encouraging message from the Bible or another inspirational book. When I was banned from going out of the house because of my poor immunity, a phone call or visitor would cheer me. Almost every time I read God's Word I came away with a word of encouragement—*almost* every time.

I trusted God to guide my decisions and to lead the medical team. Yet I admit that sometimes I wanted to call out, "Is there anyone else out there?" I had to keep reminding myself that all the seeming "coincidences" that happened just when I needed them were actually God catching me in his arms.

- In what ways do you feel as if your life is spinning out of control?
- At what times do you want to snatch your life back from the doctors, or even from God?
- How can you boost your faith in God's ability to know what's best for your life?

It's easy to encourage others to have faith. It's not so easy to live by those words yourself. Sometimes we have to make a deliberate decision to place our lives in God's hands and say, "No, there's no one else out there whom I trust. Lord, please, you take over."

**LET'S PRAY:** Lord, I hate feeling out of control. I really want to trust you, yet sometimes I want to take over and make my own decisions. Help me during those times to trust fully in you. Amen.

*The LORD will fight for you; you need only to be still.*

EXODUS 14:14

# 41

# Open My Eyes, Lord

READ: *2 Kings 6:8-17*

Elisha's servant arose early one morning and went outside. To his horror, he discovered the city where they lived had been surrounded by a great army, including horses and chariots. Filled with fear, he called Elisha. "We are doomed, sir! What shall we do?"

"Don't be afraid," Elisha answered. "We have more on our side than they have on theirs." He then prayed, "O Lord, open his eyes and let him see!" (2 Kings 6:15–17 GNT).

The Lord opened the eyes of the servant. As the man looked again, he saw hordes of horses and chariots of fire protecting them from the enemy.

The day I started radiation, I felt like that servant. I lay on the treatment bed and stared at the huge machines around me. I wanted to cry out, "Help! I'm doomed!" I saw cancer as a formidable enemy and had little confidence in the ability of those nuclear machines to rescue my body from destruction.

"Lord, show me how this is going to help," I prayed. "I'm so scared. I know the cancer cells inside my body are out of control. How can these machines help?"

I sensed a peace come over me. I knew that any cancer cells still in my body, if left alone, would multiply at a phenomenal pace. But these machines were there to wage war against them. In addition, my body's immune system was on high alert, rushing to my defense.

Cancer had declared war on my life, and from a medical point of view my future seemed bleak. But unseen by most, the Lord's soldiers had massed against the enemy. They would use these amazing machines in their fight against the truant cells. I determined to do all I could to contribute to the fight against cancer. After all, those malignant cells were already on the losing side.

- In what ways is God waging war against cancer cells in *your* body?
- Are there other forces fighting on your behalf? If you're not sure, ask the Lord to open your eyes to see them.
- Close your eyes for a moment. Can you visualize the Lord's great army massed against the cowering malignant cells?

As the radiation battle drew to an end, the fatigue became overwhelming at times. I often felt irritable and emotional. Fortunately, I'd been warned this would happen and was prepared for it. As the battle intensified, so did my determination. We would overcome. The Lord's army would see to that.

**LET'S PRAY:** Lord, I often feel overwhelmed—as if there's no hope. Yet all around me, your angels are fighting on my behalf. Help me to see you at work in my life. Thank you. Amen.

*GOD's angel sets up a circle of protection around us while we pray.*

PSALM 34:7 MESSAGE

# 42

# Lymphedema

READ: *Proverbs 2:6–11*

In addition to sharing a great deal of other information, the health visitor from Reach for Recovery emphasized the need for me to take great care of my left arm. Because several underarm lymph glands had been removed surgically, and the rest would be irradiated, I faced a risk of developing lymphedema, an abnormal swelling of my arm caused by an accumulation of lymph.

My surgeon later repeated her warning, and my oncologist detailed for me the various activities I had to avoid. "Don't carry heavy weights," they all warned. "Don't ever allow nursing staff to take your blood pressure on this arm. Nor can they use that arm to draw blood or give you intravenous therapy."

I remembered all they said and took great care to follow their instructions. I carried parcels with my right hand and only lifted light weights with my left. I didn't allow the nurses to use my left arm for any tests.

One day, Rob and I went off with our trailer for two weeks. After unhitching it from the car, we decided to push it into a better position. We both put our shoulders to the large vehicle and heaved. It rolled into position, and we set about organizing our temporary home.

That night I experienced a heavy sensation in the upper part of my left arm. By bedtime it throbbed with pain. I hardly slept.

The next morning my upper left arm was swollen, stiff, and painful. I realized how stupid I'd been. Fortunately we were only a couple of hours from town, so we set off in the car to see my doctor. He stared at me in amazement.

"You pushed a trailer? With that arm?"

Embarrassed, I muttered, "No one said I shouldn't."

"No one thought they had to!" He shook his head in obvious frustration and reached for his prescription pad. "You'll need extensive physiotherapy to prevent the lymphedema from becoming worse, and for the next couple of weeks I want you to put your arm back in the sling when you're moving around."

Although I had a few painful days, it didn't last all that long. But I learned a lesson: it wasn't enough to obey. I also needed to use my God-given intelligence.

- Why do you need to take certain precautions during this difficult time? Do you understand these measures, or do you need to ask your medical team some questions?
- What safe ways can you exercise without doing harm?
- Is there an area where you're overcautious? After that experience, I certainly was.

Sometimes we ignore the obvious in our efforts to return to normalcy. But there is also a fine line between paranoia and sensibly caring for our already overburdened bodies.

LET'S PRAY: Lord, help me differentiate between wisdom and overreaction. My body's already working overtime to cope with healing and recovery. Help me not to complicate the process. At the same time, help me to avoid becoming paranoid. Thank you, Lord. Amen.

*Wisdom can make your life pleasant and lead you safely through it.*

PROVERBS 3:17 GNT

# 43

# Where's My Harp?

**READ:** *Psalm 137:1-6*

Some years ago, a popular song spoke of hanging a harp on a weeping willow tree. The words are based on Psalm 137, where the psalmist captures the distress of the Israelites in exile. As they sat next to the rivers of Babylon, the Israelites wept as they remembered Jerusalem. They had hung up their harps. They'd given up. After all, how could they sing songs of joy in their unhappy circumstances?

They only remembered wonderful things about Jerusalem. They'd forgotten the hard times. Jerusalem was never perfect, but Babylon was worse. They were slaves. How could they sing in a foreign land?

Even though they were exiles, could it be their attitude was cutting them off from God? Was this not the very time they *needed* to sing? In all likelihood their songs would be sad, maybe confused, but at least those songs would remind them of God. They needed to lift their harps off the willow trees and show the Babylonians that they may have conquered the nation of Israel, but they hadn't conquered the spirits of her people.

Music has always played an important part in my life. My grandmother was a piano teacher, and my childhood home was full of music. By the time I left high school, I was an accomplished pianist and organist, and I soon learned to play several other instruments. I loved to have music playing in the background. When I went into the hospital, I took a portable CD player with me. All night I listened to music through earphones. It was the only way I could shut out the noises of the busy surgical ward.

When I returned home, music continued to lift my spirits. Yet I didn't play my piano. There didn't seem to be any point. I couldn't play for church because of my impaired immunity. One day I realized I needed to *make* music—not for others, for myself. I needed to remember that cancer may have attacked my body, but it couldn't touch my spirit.

- When did you last make music, either by listening to CDs or mp3s, or by playing an instrument or singing?
- How can you add more music to your life from now on?
- What music will you make today? Schedule it for a specific time so you don't forget.

The Jewish people are known for their music, both singing and dancing. When the Israelites hung up their musical instruments, they showed those around them that they'd given up. It's easy to give up in the face of cancer. But even the simple act of tuning the radio to a music program can lift our spirits and show the world "I'm not going to give up."

**LET'S PRAY:** Father, forgive me for the times I give up. Thank you for the gift of music. I pray you'll help me to draw close to you today through song and melody. Amen.

*But I will sing of your strength, in the morning I will sing of your love; for you are my fortress, my refuge in times of trouble.*

PSALM 59:16

# 44

# A Fishy Gift

READ: *Luke 12:22-31*

When I started radiation, my sister-in-law, who is a radio-therapist, warned me that toward the end of the seven weeks I would reach a point of exhaustion. "You will feel as if you can't go on," she explained. "But that means it's nearly over, so be encouraged." When I awoke on Mother's Day, I knew I'd reached that point. I didn't have the energy to get out of bed.

Later in the day, my sons breezed into my bedroom. They carried a large glass fish tank, complete with heater, pump, and other necessities. Inside swam four baby goldfish. My heart sank at the thought of the work this would involve, but I tried to look as pleased as they obviously were.

"It'll be no work at all," Stephen assured me. "The filter will keep it clean."

"It'll give you something to watch," David added. "It'll be fun." I tried to share their enthusiasm.

"This will help Mom relax," I heard my sons tell their dad. I groaned and gave a feeble smile.

As the days passed, I found the fish anything but relaxing, although they certainly gave me something to think about other than cancer. Whenever I was on my bed, I watched them closely, constantly aware of their activities. Despite being fish, they all had little personalities, and I named them accordingly. Columbus, the adventurer, caused me the most concern.

Several times every day I had to rescue him from some scrape. One day he became jammed down the side of the filter, and when I pulled him out, his beautiful gold scales were bruised. Sadly, he didn't recover, and the next day I found him floating in aimless circles. Despite extra care, he died a few hours later. I wept as I fished the intrepid little creature from the water. Jesus used birds to show how our heavenly Father cares for us. He pointed out that God supplies all their needs. He gives them shady trees, dried leaves, and animal fur to line their nests, as well as the ability to fly from one tree to the other.

- Do you have a pet that demands attention and so distracts you from your discomfort?
- When did you last sit outside or near a window and watch the birds?
- What lessons from nature tell you about God's love?

If I cared for these little fish that I hadn't even wanted in the first place, how much more God cared for me. Even when I didn't sense his presence, he was there. He knew when I needed help. No matter how tough things became, he never looked away.

**LET'S PRAY:** Loving Father, thank you for nature. Thank you for the way you care for the little creatures you made, and thank you that you care for me even more. When things get tough, please send me reminders of how much you love me. Amen.

*Look at the birds of the air; they do not sow or reap or store away in barns, and yet your heavenly Father feeds them. Are you not much more valuable than they?*

MATTHEW 6:26

# 45

# An Unlikely Neighbor

READ: *Luke 10:29–37*

A lawyer asked Jesus, "Who is my neighbor?" Jesus answered with a story.

Robbers attacked a man on an isolated road, beat him up, and left him for dead. First a priest and then a temple helper, both religious men, walked past on the other side of the road. Why? They could have been in a hurry. They may not have wanted to get dirty. Perhaps they were afraid of repercussions—the thugs still might have been in the area.

Then a Samaritan arrived on the scene. Although the Jews and Samaritans normally despised one another, this traveler ignored tradition. He tended the man's wounds, helped him onto his own donkey, and took him to an inn where someone would take care of him.

One morning I came away from radiation with a heavy heart. Rob and I were on our way to a local Indian market where I hoped to find some scarves I could fold into turbans. I was about to commence chemotherapy, and the oncologist had warned me I would lose my hair within a few days. Others who had lost their hair urged me to buy scarves, as it would be too hot to wear a wig all the time.

Before we left the hospital, I went into the cafeteria to buy juice. Behind the counter stood a Muslim lady about my age, wearing an exquisite head covering.

I blurted out, "How do you fold your scarf to look like that?"

She looked at me with compassion and asked, "Are you going to lose your hair?"

My eyes filled with tears as I nodded. The woman reached up and unraveled her turban. She spread it on the counter and spent the next few minutes teaching me what to look for and how to fold the material and fix it to my head. As I turned to leave, she placed her hand over mine and said, "I hope everything goes well."

A Muslim woman is not supposed to uncover her head in public. This lady may have faced censure in order to help me, an infidel in her culture. She would have known that I didn't embrace her beliefs, yet she showed me unquestioning love.

- What, if necessary, have you done to prepare for losing your hair?
- In what ways have you received help from an unexpected source?
- Who would be willing to help you if you asked them?

That night I practiced folding my beautiful new scarves. As I paraded them in front of my husband and sons, we laughed at the way they changed my appearance. I praised God for the Muslim lady who had been prepared to push tradition to one side and show me love.

**LET'S PRAY:** Father, thank you for the people who care more about me than about their schedules. Thank you for those who are prepared to step out of their comfort zones. Help me to be prepared to do the same for others you bring my way. Amen.

*Be kind and compassionate to one another.*

EPHESIANS 4:32

# 46

# A Good Hair Day

READ: *Matthew 6:25-32*

According to the Bible, God knew exactly how many hairs were on my head. It bothered me that soon everyone else would too. My oncologist guaranteed I would lose my hair during chemotherapy, probably after the first treatment.

Out of all the challenges I faced that year, the predicted hair loss seemed the most traumatic. For most of my life I hated my hair. At school I was called Redhead, Rusty, Ginger, Curly, and many other names. I always wished for straight, jet-black hair.

A number of people said I could expect my hair to grow back thick and beautiful. "It may even grow back another color," someone commented. Suddenly I felt satisfied with my auburn curls. I spent many minutes in prayer, pleading with the Lord to allow me to keep my hair—and I postponed getting a wig until the last moment.

The day of my first chemotherapy, another patient told us of a man who made wigs for top actresses in the country. He gave cancer patients a discount. Rob insisted we go to see him.

The man sat me down and ran his fingers through my hair, studying it professionally. He left the room and returned moments later with an attractive red box. He smiled brightly at my reflection in the mirror.

"Close your eyes, and don't open them again until I say so," he instructed.

I squeezed my eyes shut as dread filled my mind. I felt my head being encased in a snug-fitting cap, followed by a few deft touches. Then he said, "Please open your eyes."

Apprehensively, I looked into the mirror. The woman who stared back at me could have been my identical twin sister. I drew in a sharp breath. Rob gasped. The man beamed. The wig was a perfect match and brought healing to my traumatized emotions.

It was fine that God would know how many hairs lurked beneath the wig, but I felt reassured that I wouldn't have to "walk naked" if all my hair fell out—and yes, I was still praying it wouldn't.

- Can you imagine counting every hair on your head? Or is that real easy at the moment?
- How do you think the Lord feels when he sees you lose your hair?
- If your little girl had to go through this difficult experience, would you not want to hold her close and assure her of your love? Your heavenly Father longs to do the same for you.

That day I learned another important lesson: it's not vanity to try to make yourself look and feel better. Wash your hair (if you have any). Put on some makeup, wear bright clothes, and force a smile. You'll be surprised at the difference these things make to your emotions. By the way, I never got to wear that wig. The Lord answered my prayer. My hair wouldn't have taken any prizes at a beauty salon, but it didn't fall out and it didn't change color.

**LET'S PRAY:** Lord, forgive me when I panic over matters I can't control. Help me to know when to keep praying and when to accept the situation and move forward. Thank you that you gave me every hair on my head, even when I can count them on my fingers. Thank you for loving me so much, with or without hair. Amen.

*Even the hairs on your head are counted.*

MATTHEW 10:30 CEV

# 47

## What Do I Want?

READ: *Mark 10:46-52*

A blind beggar at the side of the road cried out for help. Jesus called him closer and asked, "What do you want me to do for you?"

How ridiculous. That was a silly question for Jesus to ask. Or was it? Did the beggar have ulterior motives? Did he want to trap Jesus into displaying his miraculous power?

Just a short time before, Jesus had asked two of his disciples the same question: "What do you want me to do for you?" They had replied in a way that showed they were seeking power and prestige.

Bartimaeus, the beggar, thought before he answered. Would Jesus heal him? Or would he, Bartimaeus, get into trouble with those who didn't understand his motives? He only had one desire: he wanted his sight. It was humanly impossible, but at that moment the blind man seemed to know Jesus could work a miracle.

Often during times of prayer I tussled with this same question. What did I really want the Lord to do for me? I knew what I wanted. I wanted never to have had cancer. But it was too late for that. So what should I ask?

Several times doctors assured me that many people who went through radiation and chemotherapy lived for at least five years after the cancer was removed. But I didn't want five more years. I wanted to live and be fit. I wanted to grow old and watch my grandchildren grow up. I needed a miracle.

I thought long and hard about the story of Bartimaeus, then came to a decision. "Lord," I prayed, "you know what I want. I want to make a full recovery. I want to live a fruitful life. Please heal me in such a way that others will glorify you."

- If Jesus were to stand in front of you today, what do you think he would ask you?
- How would you answer his question, "What do you want me to do for you?"
- What prevents you from asking for a miracle?

I longed to receive healing, yet I held back from asking. After all, how would I know I'd been healed? Many times people suggested I should have faith and refuse treatment. Two people I knew said that the Lord had healed them. They both stopped treatment, and I played the organ at their funerals. I knew I could stop treatment only if *God* showed me that I was completely and miraculously healed. It wasn't a matter of faith. It was being realistic. The only way I could have known for sure I'd been healed was if the surgeon had operated and found the tumor already gone. I knew God could have done this, but he hadn't. So I decided to pray for healing, then persevere with the medical treatment.

It wasn't easy, and there were a number of times I felt like giving up, but today I give thanks for the miracles God performed in my life as a result of medical science.

**LET'S PRAY:** Lord Jesus, I wish this cancer had never happened, but please help me through this difficult time. Please give me my health back in your time and in your way. Amen.

*Jesus said to her, "I am the resurrection and the life. The one who believes in me will live, even though they die; and whoever lives by believing in me will never die. Do you believe this?"*

JOHN 11:25–26

# 48

## Write It Down

READ: *Jeremiah 30:1-3*

It was my first day of chemotherapy. I had heard many horror stories of people who started to vomit before they even got home. It took me an hour to get from the oncologist to the house, and yet I felt great.

It had been a long and stressful day, so I climbed on the bed and lay with my eyes closed. Minutes later, I jerked them open. Why was I lying there doing nothing? I felt wonderful. Although I had a journal at my bedside, I hadn't written in it for weeks. I sat up in bed and wrote, "Chemo—Day 1: I feel great." I slipped off the bed and went to see how Rob was getting on with supper. The oncologist had given me tablets to take the moment I started to feel ill, yet I was looking forward to a good meal.

The intravenous cortisone the oncologist administered with the chemotherapy drugs gave me an emotional and physical boost. I soon found that, for me, the best day of each chemotherapy cycle was always the day of treatment.

Several times a day, I made a quick note in my journal. I didn't try to pretend. If I felt dreadful, I said so. I wrote it clearly, so that I could read it at a glance. I soon came to appreciate the value of this practice. It helped me plan my days. I could look back at previous treatment cycles and predict which days I could expect to feel well and which days I was likely to spend in isolation because of my dangerously low cell count.

Throughout Scripture, God kept telling his people to "write it down." Not only did God want to ensure that all the people would hear the message, he also wanted historical records. The people I read about in the Bible were far from perfect, yet they faithfully told of their experiences and their reactions so I could learn from them. As I read of their shortcomings, I was encouraged. If God carried them through their many crises, I felt sure he would do the same for me.

- Why do you think God would want you to remember what's happening in your life at the moment?
- What short notes can you write today that may help you in the future?
- Have you read any books or notes written by people who have traveled the cancer journey? If not, ask your friends to find you something to read with a positive message.*

My records not only helped me cope with the days immediately ahead, they also formed a base for me in the future. As I reread my entries, I saw God's hand upon my life. Years later, when I started to write about my experiences, I could check my journal for facts. God was indeed good—and I have records to prove it.

**LET'S PRAY:** Lord God, you've helped me through so many situations. I can't see how I could ever forget them, but time is a healer, and I might. So please help me write what I need to remember. Amen.

*Then the LORD replied: "Write down the revelation and make it plain on tablets so that a herald may run with it."*

HABAKKUK 2:2

---

*See appendix 2 on page 203 for a few suggestions.

# 49

## Learning the Hard Way

READ: *Joshua 2:12-19*

When I started chemotherapy, my oncologist said, "Whenever your white cell count is low, you are not to mix with people. Especially on days three, four, and five, when your immunity will be especially low. You are not to go out of the house during those days, understand?" I nodded my head.

That was Thursday. Sunday was day four, and I looked as bad as I felt. When Rob saw me getting dressed for church, he reminded me of the oncologist's instructions. I shook my head in defiance.

"No one stops me from going to church. I'll be careful."

I promised to sit with friends who would take me home if necessary. I also sat at the front, away from the main congregation—mistake number one. It was winter, and the congregation, with all their cold and flu germs, sat behind me. I would have been safer at the back. During the service I became really ill and knew I'd been foolish. I also realized the house keys were in my husband's pocket, and he was preaching. So I couldn't go home.

I should have learned a lesson from Rahab in the Old Testament. The Israelites were about to invade the Promised Land. Joshua sent two spies into Jericho, the first major city, to reconnoiter and bring back vital information. If it hadn't been for Rahab, a known prostitute, they would have been captured and killed. In return for their safety, the men agreed to protect Rahab and her family when the Israelite army attacked the city.

"Hang a rope of scarlet thread from the window," the men instructed. "But make sure everyone is inside the house. We will not be responsible for anyone who goes out of the house once the raid commences."

When the army attacked, Rahab obeyed instructions. All of her family members who took refuge in her home were saved. I'm sure some of them wanted to flee. If they had followed their own inclinations, they would have died. Their obedience gave them salvation.

As a result of my refusal to follow instructions, I spent eight days fighting for my life in a sterile isolation ward of the hospital.

- What instruction don't you understand or do you want to rebel against?
- During which days in your treatment cycle do you need to be extra careful of your health?
- When are you tempted to go your own way if you don't like the restrictions? Better check with the Lord (and your doctor) first!

God wanted Rahab to stay in her home so he could protect her. Likewise, there were times during my treatment when I had to stay in my home. When I stopped rebelling, God met with me there and I had many special times alone with him.

**LET'S PRAY:** Father, I'm a social being. It's so hard to isolate myself. Help me to see the times when I cannot be with other people as opportunities for special fellowship with you. Amen.

*If you keep my commands, you will remain in my love, just as I have kept my Father's commands and remain in his love.*

JOHN 15:10

# 50

## My Will Be Done

READ: *Luke 22:39–44*

I refuse to go to the hospital." Tears streamed down my cheeks. "I want to go home to my own bed."

The oncologist ignored me as he continued to make arrangements over the phone for my immediate hospitalization into a sterile isolation ward. He put the phone down and looked at my husband. "Take her directly to the oncology ward at the hospital. Do *not* go to the admissions office. She must get into isolation as quickly as possible. The nurses on the ward are expecting her."

I pulled myself to my feet with difficulty and tried to ignore my wobbly knees. "I said I'm not going to the hospital." I think I would have stamped my feet if I'd had the strength.

"Don't go home to fetch anything," the oncologist repeated, still speaking to Rob. "I'll be there to see her in about an hour."

I continued to weep and didn't say good-bye. Rob took my elbow and steered me through the rain. I trudged through muddy puddles on our way to the car.

As Rob started the engine, I blurted out, "Forget what he said. Take me home. I will *not* go to the hospital." I sounded like a petulant child, but I was too ill to care. Rob swung the car in the direction of the hospital and drove without saying a word. I cried. I begged. My husband continued to drive. I curled myself into a fetal position against the car door and cradled my muddy right foot on my left thigh. Tears flowed down my cheeks. No one understood. No one cared. They seemed to forget—this was my life, not theirs.

By the time I arrived in the ward, common sense and good manners prevailed. I clambered onto the sterile white bed and said a tearful good-bye to Rob. For the next two hours I tried to ignore the muddy footprint on my cream linen slacks until my family managed to bring my pajamas.

A couple of days later, I read the story of Jesus on his way to the cross. He left the upper room with his disciples and made his way to the Garden of Gethsemane, knowing what awaited him. He also wept, as he prayed in the garden. He pleaded with his Father that he wouldn't need to go through the ordeal that lay ahead. Yet that's where the similarities ended. Jesus added, "Not my will, however, but your will be done" (Luke 22:42 GNT).

Jesus trusted his heavenly Father to know best.

- When have you reacted in panic? Did you make wise decisions?
- What part of your treatment is most difficult for you? What plan can you make to help yourself cope?
- How do you feel about praying, "Not my will but yours be done"?

**LET'S PRAY:** Father, help me to trust you no matter what I face. Give me courage for the difficult times, and help me to behave in a way that others will know I belong to you. Amen.

*Father, if you are willing, take this cup from me; yet not my will, but yours be done.*

LUKE 22:42

# 51

## God, Where Are You?

READ: *Psalm 22:1-5*

I lay alone in the isolation room. My friends were not allowed to visit. My husband had gone home, and my sons were at work. I felt abandoned by everyone, even by God. I had always believed he would never leave me, but where was he now?

I lay on the sterile sheets and felt a wave of terror. The expression on my oncologist's face when he read my blood count results told me of his concern. I had seen the look of horror on the senior nurse's face when I shuffled into the ward, having refused the wheelchair that awaited my arrival at the hospital. I knew my condition was critical.

So where was God? Had he forgotten me? Maybe I just wasn't good enough. I had been a Christian for many years, but perhaps now that I'd reached the end, I didn't measure up.

Fighting tears, I glanced around the room and spotted a Bible. I flipped it open and started to read Psalm 22.

David, the great king whom God called "a man after his own heart" (1 Sam. 13:14) faced tremendous suffering with no apparent relief from God. His enemies surrounded him like a pack of hyenas. Helpless and exhausted, he cried to God, "Why have you forsaken me?" (Ps. 22:1).

Hundreds of years later, Jesus, God's own Son, echoed those words as he hung on that dreadful cross (Matt. 27:46). I lay back on the hard white pillow. David and Jesus both felt abandoned by God. I was in good company. I knew that God did not fail David or Jesus. Peace washed over me as I realized that, lonely though I felt, God would not fail me either.

- When, if ever, have you felt isolated from friends or family?
- What, if anything, causes you to feel as if God has abandoned you?
- If you feel far from God, who's moved—you or him?

It's not a sin to feel depressed; nor is it wrong to feel abandoned, even by God. Cancer causes your emotions to swing, but be assured that although your feelings may change, God's love is changeless. When we find ourselves far from him, he's not the one who's moved. He will never abandon his children.

**LET'S PRAY:** Lord God, sometimes I feel so alone. Thank you for your promise that nothing can separate me from your love. Help me to trust you in spite of my feelings. Amen.

*Do not be far from me, for trouble is near and there is no one to help.*

PSALM 22:11

# 52

# Skateboarding

**READ:** *Proverbs 3:1–12*

"Wakey wakey!" The cheery wake-up call shattered my deep sleep.

After the nurses had performed their usual early morning tests, I eased myself out of the high hospital bed and leaned on my IV stand for support. I shuffled to the bathroom and closed the door behind me. I ran myself a bath, clumsily removed my clothes, and threaded them over the drip tubing. I eased myself over the edge of the white tub and sank with relief into the warm water, taking care not to wet the bandage that secured the IV needle in place above my right breast.

When I'd finished bathing, I pulled myself to my feet and gripped the IV stand. I placed one foot over the edge of the tub and onto the slatted wooden bath-rack. As I transferred my weight onto the slats, the rack took on a life of its own. It careened recklessly toward the door. I balanced on one leg and clung to the IV stand as it skated wildly across the wet tiles.

It's amazing how much your mind can process in seconds. My overwhelming fear was that the stand would fall over. I imagined the needle wrenched from the port that led directly to my heart. I had brief but realistic visions of a blood-spattered bathroom.

In my attempt to keep the metal stand upright, I pirouetted across the bathroom until the wheels of the IV stand cannoned into the door. I overbalanced, fell backward, and finally came to rest on my side, with the stand still erect. Shaken, I lay for a moment, then untangled myself from the tubing. I rose unsteadily to my feet, pulled on my fresh clothes, and made my way gingerly back to bed, bruised but intact—and still hanging on to my IV stand.

King Solomon, known as the wisest man who ever lived, recognized that as God's children we will go through rough patches. There will be times when we can't see how we'll survive. We may come out feeling bruised, but as long as we hang on for dear life to our God, he will see us through.

- Do you feel as if you're sliding out of control? What's the cause?
- What can you do today to hang on to God?
- When has God been there for you, even when things seemed desperate?

If I hadn't been so concerned about my drip, the fall might have been much worse. The panic that I would pull the needle from my chest saved me from what could have been serious injury. There are times when everything seems to go crazy. We're not able to think clearly. That's when we need to hang on to God for dear life. He will not let us go.

**LET'S PRAY:** Father, thank you that even when things seem to slide out of control, you are still there. Help me to remember your promises and hang on to you no matter what happens. Amen.

*Even though I walk through the darkest valley, I will fear no evil, for you are with me; your rod and your staff, they comfort me.*

PSALM 23:4

# 53

## Hit the Dirt!

READ: *Psalm 40:11–13*

I lay in the sterile isolation ward with my white cell count nearly zero. My immune system had reached critical levels. My husband and sons were only allowed to visit if they donned gowns, masks, and gloves before entering the room. The nursing staff and even the custodians had to dress the same way.

One night the nurse in charge rushed into my room to give me my medication. She was obviously upset and flustered. A bottle slipped from her fingers and pills scattered across the floor. In tears, she knelt to pick them up. I slid from my bed and joined her on the floor. I crawled around picking up pills until we collected them all. She then helped me back into bed as I was too weak to get off the floor on my own.

Late that night, I lay in the darkened ward and thought over this incident.

"How incredibly stupid!" I muttered. "Of all the places—crawling on the floor." I hadn't even washed my hands before I got back in bed.

I wondered if the nurse gave this another thought. How could she have allowed a patient with a dangerously low white cell count to crawl around on the floor? If I had told the day staff, the girl probably would have lost her job. However, the Lord remained in control and I suffered no harm. From that moment on, I tried to remember how ill I was and behaved accordingly. Still, for those few minutes it had been nice to do something helpful for someone else.

As I read Psalm 40:2 (below), I imagined the Lord stretching down and lifting me off the germ-laden floor and setting me safely back on my bed. How good to know his protection.

- What occasions can you think of when you did something foolish but the Lord protected you?
- What precautions do you take from germs and infection when your blood count is low?
- How good is it to know that when you are careless, the Lord doesn't give up on you?

During treatment it is exceedingly important that we safeguard our health and avoid any risk of contamination or contact with infection. We don't need to be paranoid, but we do need to be careful. At the same time, it is good to remember that healing ultimately comes from God.

**LET'S PRAY:** Lord God, thank you for the marvels of the human body. Even though cancer is such a devastating enemy, you have given my body resilience and an ability to fight back that amazes me. Help me to play my part in this fight, never forgetting that you are in control. Amen.

*He lifted me out of the slimy pit, out of the mud and mire; he set my feet on a rock and gave me a firm place to stand.*

PSALM 40:2

# 54

# New Every Morning

READ: *Lamentations 3:19-26*

In one of the well-loved *Peanuts* cartoons, Linus says to Charlie Brown, "Life is difficult, isn't it, Charlie Brown?"

Charlie replies, "Yes, it is. But I've developed a new philosophy. I only dread one day at a time."

After a week in isolation, I was thrilled when the oncologist allowed me to leave the room for brief periods and walk down the corridor. I was not so thrilled when he said he planned to give me the next dose of chemotherapy the following morning. I lay awake that night, dreading a repeat of the same drama and wondering if I would survive.

In the Sermon on the Mount, Jesus pointed out that one day has all the problems we can cope with. We can't live tomorrow today. We don't have the strength, the courage, or even the faith to deal with the future. God promises to give us strength for *today*. When tomorrow comes, then he will supply what we need to get us through the challenges of that day too.

- What worries you about your future?
- Is there something specific that you dread about the coming weeks or months?
- Do you have a book of cartoons or some funny videos you can enjoy? If not, who can you ask to get you one?

As it was, my worrying was a waste of energy. The oncologist dropped the dosage of medication, and I had no severe reactions from that round of chemo. Twenty-four hours after the treatment, he discharged me from the hospital. How often do we allow ourselves to imagine the worst, especially when it comes to chemotherapy, instead of trusting the Lord?

**LET'S PRAY:** Lord God, thank you for bringing me this far. You know the worries and fears I have for the future. Help me to live for today—and trust you to give me the strength I'll need, when I need it. Thank you. Amen.

*Because of the* LORD's *great love we are not consumed, for his compassions never fail. They are new every morning; great is your faithfulness.*

LAMENTATIONS 3:22–23

# 55

## Is There a Future?

**READ:** *Psalm 118:5-8, 17*

It was day three after my latest chemo treatment, which meant my white cell count was near zero. My almost nonexistent immunity meant I couldn't mix with people. I lay back on my bed and allowed waves of self-pity to wash over me. My husband and sons had left for church and wouldn't be home for a couple of hours. It took all my energy to heave myself into a sitting position against the pillows. Tears burned my eyes and ran down my cheeks.

After a few minutes, I made a halfhearted attempt to pull myself together. I turned on the radio next to the bed in the hope that I would find a Christian sermon. I did—in Afrikaans, a language I knew and understood but that required more concentration than I felt capable of.

Disgusted, I clicked it off and reached for my Bible. I flicked it open and focused on the first words I saw: "I will not die but live, and will proclaim what the LORD has done" (Ps. 118:17).

I felt a leap of encouragement and excitement. I wasn't about to die. Not right then, anyway. Not until I had the opportunity to tell others what the Lord had done for me.

I would like to say from that moment on I never felt sorry for myself, but that would be a lie. However, I never forgot that promise. I started to list in my journal all the things I would tell people when—not if—I survived. My mind-set changed as I looked for things I could share with my visitors.

- What makes you feel sorry for yourself?
- When you read Psalm 139:7–8 (below), how does it make you feel?
- How often do you ask the Lord to speak to you before reading from his Word?

Sometimes it seems as if cancer treatment does us more harm than good. As our physical state weakens, our emotions plummet. We look like death, and our feelings follow. Praise God for his Word and for the way he makes individual verses come alive to us at moments such as this. Words that we normally would skim over bring us a message from the living God. "You will . . . proclaim what the Lord has done"—those were his words to me fifteen years ago. What are his words for you today?

**LET'S PRAY:** Lord, I'm tired of feeling so ill. I long for some words of encouragement. Please speak to me today and open my ears that I may hear you. Amen.

*Where can I go from your Spirit? Where can I flee from your presence? If I go up to the heavens, you are there; if I make my bed in the depths, you are there.*

PSALM 139:7–8

# 56

# Journaling with God

READ: *1 Samuel 3:1-10*

One morning as I tried to read my Bible, I couldn't concentrate. Thoughts crowded out the words. Eventually I reached for my journal, picked up a pen, and wrote to the Lord.

"How long is this going to go on? I long to hear your voice. What does the future hold?"

Into my mind came words, and I continued to write. "You cannot see your future. I will show you all you need to know in good time. Trust me with your future. I am already there."

I sat back, puzzled. I realized those were not my words. The Lord had spoken to me. With a sense of excitement, I wrote another question. Sure enough, more words came to mind. I wrote them down as fast as I could. My feelings of aloneness faded as I held a dialogue on paper with the Lord.

Samuel was about twelve when he first heard from God. Like me, he had to learn to listen. Because of a promise his mother made before he was born, Samuel lived in the tabernacle and worked with Eli, the aging priest. While Eli slept in a separate room, Samuel slept inside the sanctuary itself.

One night after Samuel lay down to sleep, a voice broke through his thoughts. "Samuel, Samuel."

He called out, "I'm here!" then jumped up and went to Eli.

"I didn't call you," the old man said. "Go back to bed."

No sooner was Samuel back in bed than the voice came again. "Samuel, Samuel!"

Once again he went to Eli.

"I didn't call you," the priest repeated. "Go back to bed."

The third time this happened, the old man realized it must be the Lord calling the boy. "Go back to bed," he said, "and if the voice comes again say, 'Speak Lord, for your servant is listening.'" Samuel went back to bed and did as instructed. When the Lord spoke again, Samuel replied to God and then listened.

- Has the Lord ever spoken to you in a clear way? Do you expect him to?
- If he speaks, how will you remember what he says?
- Have you ever written a letter to God? If not, try it. You may be surprised.

So often our prayers are one-sided, and we wonder why God doesn't speak to us. We need to say, "Speak Lord, for I am listening." Then we must keep quiet—and listen.

**LET'S PRAY:** Lord, I long to hear your voice, yet I so seldom listen. Help me to follow Samuel's example and eagerly pay attention. Please speak to me and teach me how to listen. Amen.

*My dear brothers and sisters, take note of this: Everyone should be quick to listen, slow to speak and slow to become angry.*

JAMES 1:19

# 57

# I Can't Go On

READ: *Exodus 18:13-24*

One day when I went to the laboratory for blood tests, I learned they had decided to terminate my employment. "It's the only way we can take on someone else in your place," my about-to-be ex-boss explained. "But the moment you are well enough, we'll open a vacancy for you."

When I returned home, I sat and stared out the window. *It's not worth the struggle*, I thought. Then I remembered my family and all the incomplete projects in my life, and I knew I couldn't give up.

At times like these, I made the effort to be honest with God. He already knew how I felt, so why pretend? If I had to have cancer, at least he could deal with my side effects faster.

"Lord, please push up my white cell count," I would cry. "I'm trying to be brave, but I don't feel as if I can carry on. Show me what you expect me to do."

The answer often came not in the miraculous way I wanted, but through my inability to do anything but relax on my bed or in an armchair. God knew what I needed better than any doctor. He wanted me to rest. He often sent me visitors with words of encouragement or prompted me to read a book with a message that edified me. When I was too tired to keep going, God showed me what I needed to do.

In the Old Testament we read of how the great prophet Moses also reached a point of exhaustion. God had used him in a mighty way to lead his people out of Egypt. He had faced the evil Pharaoh not once, but many times. He had seen God work amazing miracles, like the time he divided the Red Sea. But Moses was tired. All day long he sat and listened to people's problems.

Jethro, his father-in-law, came to visit and rejoiced in all the Lord was doing for the people. But the next day, after he'd watched Moses at work, he came to his son-in-law.

"This is no good!" he said. He instructed Moses to delegate the workload so that he could get some rest. "This is way too much for you," he said. "You can't do this alone" (Exod. 18:18 Message).

- What causes you to be exhausted or disheartened?
- If God were to speak to you right now, what do you think he would say?
- How would you reply?

We so often take on more than we can cope with. I hate to do nothing, and even when I was trying to survive cancer treatment, I wanted to keep busy. But that's not always the best policy. The Lord doesn't expect us to push ourselves beyond our limits. Sometimes we have to allow ourselves extra rest. Healing will come as God strengthens us through times of rest and through the encouragement of those who care for us.

**LET'S PRAY:** Lord, you know how I feel right now. Show me how to care for my body and mind. Help me to get past this hurdle. Please lift my spirits, Lord. Amen.

*For in six days the LORD made the heavens and the earth, the sea, and all that is in them, but he rested on the seventh day.*

EXODUS 20:11

# 58

# Help My Unbelief!

**READ:** *Matthew 17:14-20*

I hung on to the words I had recently read in Scripture—"I will not die but live, and will proclaim what the LORD has done" (Ps. 118:17). I truly believed God had led me to that passage.

So if I believed his words, how come I was sometimes afraid to fall asleep? Why did I wonder if I would die before morning? And so what if I did? Why was I afraid? As a Christian of many years, I had counseled a number of people that if they truly put their faith in the Lord Jesus, they need never fear death. Yet here I was, fighting to stay alive.

"Lord," I cried out, following the pattern of prayer given by an anxious father so long ago, "I do have faith. But please help me to have more."

The father had brought his son to Jesus. The boy suffered from epilepsy, and his fits were so violent the father feared for his life. The man pleaded with Jesus for help, saying, "If you can do anything, take pity on us and help us" (Mark 9:22).

Jesus replied, "Why do you say 'if you can'? Anything is possible for someone who has faith!" (Mark 9:23 CEV).

"I do have faith," the boy's father cried out. "Please help me to have even more" (9:24).

In the past I had wondered about this man's words. Surely, either you had faith or you didn't. But now I understood the man's dilemma. So I prayed that same prayer.

Yes, I believed Jesus could heal me. Yes, I believed the power of God was way greater than the power of cancer. But intellectually I struggled. Why would he heal *me*?

I had known others who died of cancer. Well-meaning people avoided my eyes as they reminded me that "God can do all things." Unbelief crept in and caused me to doubt. What if I did die? I knew I would go straight to heaven to be with the Lord. I believed that to my core, and yet I didn't want to die.

- When you look at your treatment schedule, what are you most afraid of?
- Do you know for sure that you'll go to heaven one day? If so, then what causes you to fear?*
- What's the best thing about going to heaven?

I came to understand that God wanted me to fight death because it wasn't my time to die. He had other plans for me. I had faith, but I needed to keep fighting. I have since watched others leave this earthly life to go home to the Lord. They didn't fight; they had peace. It was their time.

We never need to fear death. We only need to be ready. God will take care of the rest when our time comes. In the meantime, all things are possible.

**LET'S PRAY:** Lord, thank you for the assurance of heaven when I die. Give me the faith to hang on as long as you want me here on earth. And when the time comes for me to go home, reassure me with your perfect peace. Thank you, Lord. Amen.

*But when you ask, you must believe and not doubt, because the one who doubts is like a wave of the sea, blown and tossed by the wind.*

JAMES 1:6

*If you're not sure, please read "New Relationship" on p. 192.

# 59

## Forever in Sight

READ: *Psalm 139:9-12*

One Monday morning we woke early to the promise of a beautiful African summer day. It was Rob's day off, and we planned to get away from the house for a break.

"Let's go to the botanical gardens," Rob suggested.

The Walter Sisulu Botanical Gardens were a half hour drive from our home and one of our favorite hangouts. We walked through the stone archway, paid our entrance fees, and meandered hand-in-hand along the paved path. We passed signposts showing the way to the bird and butterfly garden, the cycad garden, and the forest walk. I lacked the energy to follow all the possible routes, so we took the most direct path to our main objective, the waterfall.

On either side of the path, rich green lawn encouraged us to throw off our shoes and enjoy the feel of the soft, luxuriant grass. We strained our eyes to spot the cuckoo whose melodic call followed us, but it remained hidden from view. We stopped frequently to admire the vast variety of indigenous shrubs and bushes. Butterflies flitted among the flowers clustered in stunning displays. From a distance, the sound of rushing water beckoned us.

Eventually we came to the spectacular waterfall, which is the most popular scenic attraction of these magnificent gardens. Water splashed down the steep cliff into a rock pool. We sat on the stone wall and focused our binoculars on a spot near the top of the cliff, searching for the aerie where the garden's pair of Verreaux's eagles nested.

"Look, there he is!" Rob exclaimed.

High above us, an eagle soared with wings outstretched. Although we couldn't make out its features, I knew the bird could spot a rabbit from a mile away, so it could certainly see us. It continued to soar overhead, unperturbed by any activities in the valley below.

We spread a rug on the well-manicured lawn and unpacked our picnic lunch. I had heard of young eagles mistaking plastic bottles for fish. I hoped the large bird hovering above was old enough to tell the difference between fish and our bottles of fruit juice!

While that eagle may have had incredible vision, it would eventually lose sight of me if it kept soaring. I remembered the words of Psalm 139, and I knew that with God it is different. No matter how far from God I might feel, he never takes his eyes off me.

- At what times have you been conscious of God watching over you?
- How can you improve your awareness of God?
- When are you especially grateful for God's never-ceasing supervision?

How good to know that even if I *tried* to hide from God, he would always be able to see me. His sight is better than any eagle's.

**LET'S PRAY:** Father God, thank you for the lessons we can learn from the eagle. Thank you for the assurance that no matter how bad things may seem, you are always there watching over me. Help me to see you at work in my life. Amen.

*The eyes of the Lord are everywhere, keeping watch.*

PROVERBS 15:3

# 60

## Lousy Timing

READ: *Matthew 6:19-21*

B ye," I called to Rob as I headed for the car on the way for blood tests.

Rob pushed back his chair. "You're not up to driving today, Shirl. I'll take you."

We went out the back door and locked it behind us, leaving our three dogs in the backyard. We were gone half an hour.

When we returned, I found the dogs agitated, and I soon saw why.

The front door had been jimmied off its hinges. Our TV was gone, as were the VCR, the microwave, and many other items. The shelves of the linen cupboard stood empty. The dogs had heard the intruders, but they were locked out of the house and powerless to do anything.

My first reaction was to say to Rob, "Oh no. What lousy timing. You should have let me go alone. Then this wouldn't have happened. They must have been watching the house."

When the police arrived, the constable in charge corrected me.

"There is a gang operating in this suburb at present. They take the people by surprise and tie them up, then rob the house at leisure." He held up a coil of green twine. "We found this in the garden. It was meant for you two. Be grateful that your husband wasn't home when they arrived."

After they left, Rob and I took stock. We had lost a number of material items, but they could be replaced. Neither of us had been injured or killed. We praised the Lord that he had watched over us with such perfect timing.

Jesus warned his followers not to fuss over material possessions. He said, "Do not store up riches for yourselves here on earth, where . . . robbers break in and steal" (Matt. 6:19 GNT). He urged his listeners not to worry about their future but to take life one day at a time.

I thought of my cancer struggle. There were many activities I could no longer enjoy. I had lost my job. My clothes no longer fit, and my hair and skin looked dreadful. But these were all temporary issues. One day I'd look back and see God's timing as perfect.

- Do you feel as if your cancer occurred at an inopportune time?
- Think about it: Would there really have been a better time?
- When has God intervened at just the right moment?

There is never a convenient time to have cancer. Yet your cancer didn't catch God by surprise. He watches over you all the time. He's standing by you right this minute. Speak to him and tell him how you feel.

**LET'S PRAY:** Lord God, you know this cancer has come at a lousy time in my life. I never wanted it, but certainly not now. Show me how to live my life one day at a time, and help me to treasure the things that matter and let go of those that don't. Amen.

*Therefore do not worry about tomorrow, for tomorrow will worry about itself. Each day has enough trouble of its own.*

MATTHEW 6:34

# 61

## Not the Way I Expected

READ: *Acts 12:1-17*

Often God didn't seem to hear my prayers. "Please help my blood count not to drop this time." The next day it was lower than ever.

"Don't let the oncologist give me chemo this week. I'm not over the last one." I had the chemo.

"Please let me be well enough to go to church on Sunday." Surely he would answer *that* prayer. I awoke too sick to go to church.

At times like these, it was easy to forget the prayers he *did* answer. Like the time my oncologist agreed to postpone my treatment so I could attend my youngest son's graduation. "On the condition that your blood count is above four," he added. My cell count was so high the pathologist checked it twice.

Then there was Christmas. We had reservations at an upscale restaurant for Christmas dinner. I was afraid I would be too ill to go, but not only did I get there, I even enjoyed the meal.

Sometimes God didn't answer the way I expected and I nearly missed the answer. Like the time I prayed for a special friend to walk through cancer with me—and he gave me a stuffed lion (see "A Lion-Sized Gift," p. 48). And like the time I asked for help in finding a suitable headscarf, and he gave me "An Unlikely Neighbor" (see p. 102).

In the book of Acts, we read how wicked King Herod arrested the disciple James and had him put to death. He then threw Peter into jail. The church prayed fervently for his safety.

The night before Peter's trial, a group from the church gathered in a home to pray. Time was running out. How they prayed for Peter! Would God intervene? Or would Peter be put to death? Suddenly they heard someone knocking on the door. They continued to pray as a servant girl, Rhoda, went to answer it. Moments later she barged into the prayer meeting.

"Peter is here!" she exclaimed in excitement.

"You're out of your mind," they told her.

No doubt someone asked, "Where is he then?"

"I left him outside," she must have replied. She was so thrilled when she heard Peter's voice that she ran to tell the others without letting him into the house. I can imagine Rhoda's sheepish expression as she waited for their reaction. When they saw she really believed it was Peter, they came to the conclusion that it was his ghost. And the whole time poor Peter remained outside, knocking on the door.

Eventually they opened the door and—surprise!—Peter was there. God answered their prayers—but not the way they had expected. And they nearly missed the answer.

- When did you receive an unexpected answer to your prayers?
- What prayers, if any, does God not seem to have heard?
- Where are you looking for the answers?

God doesn't mind when I ask for his help, but I need to trust his judgment on how he answers. After all, that's why he's God and I'm not.

**LET'S PRAY:** Loving Father, thank you for all the prayers you answer. Teach me to look eagerly for the answers, however you choose to send them. Amen.

*Nothing is impossible for God.*

LUKE 1:37 CEV

135

# 62

## I Need You

READ: *Mark 14:37–41*

Many times I craved company, yet people couldn't always drop what they were doing to be with me. My husband had services to prepare for and a congregation to care for. My daughter, Debbie, lived halfway across the world. My elder son lived in a nearby town, and David, my youngest, had just started his first job. Sometimes, in the early hours of the morning, loneliness or fear crept in. My husband needed his sleep. If only I had someone to keep me company. I wanted to call out, "Somebody, help! I need you!"

Jesus knew that feeling. On the night of his arrest, he and his disciples ate supper together. After Judas Iscariot left to betray the Lord, Jesus and the remaining eleven disciples walked down the slopes of the Mount of Olives.

When they arrived in the Garden of Gethsemane, Jesus said to his disciples, "Stay here and keep watch with me."

The full realization of what lay ahead seemed to have become a reality to Jesus. He knew he was about to sacrifice his life as payment for sins he hadn't committed. He faced rejection by the people who had witnessed his many miracles and heard his teachings. His best friends would forsake him. And worst—God would turn his back on his Son. That night, Jesus did not want to be alone.

- When do you most often long for company?
- What does it mean to you that you can call on Jesus at any time of the day or night?

- Is there someone who perhaps needs *your* prayer support and encouragement? Sometimes the best way to have a friend is to be one.

I found comfort in the knowledge that the Lord knew and understood my need for companionship. At least I had him. I knew Jesus would never let me down—unlike the disciples, who failed him in his time of need.

**LET'S PRAY:** Lord, I need you to watch with me right now. Please stay close. Amen.

*Watch and pray so that you will not fall into temptation. The spirit is willing, but the flesh is weak.*

MARK 14:38

# 63

# A Tough Decision

READ: *Luke 9:51-62*

Every few weeks, dread filled my heart when I headed toward my next chemotherapy treatment. It was all I could do to keep from saying, "Stop the car! Turn around. Take me home."

I remember one time in particular. I had just recovered from a particularly severe reaction to the previous chemotherapy, and I was on my way for another treatment. "I can't believe I'm doing this," I muttered to my husband, trying to quell my inner panic. "I'm deliberately subjecting my body to more of the drugs that made me so ill last time. This is crazy."

"No, not crazy," my husband replied. "You're doing it for the future. Just think, only four more treatments and you'll get your life back."

That day, as I allowed the cytotoxic liquid to run into my veins, I thought of Jesus on the way to Calvary. Scripture says, "He stedfastly set his face to go to Jerusalem" (Luke 9:51 KJV). Despite knowing what lay ahead, Jesus made up his mind and committed himself to the journey.

Ahead lay many trials, disappointments, and frustrations. He would still give much teaching, perform many miracles, and change numerous lives, yet he knew his time was short. He determined to make the most of what was left. Nothing would dissuade him from going forward, despite the knowledge that he faced a time of torment, suffering, and ultimately death.

Jesus knew that after the horror of the crucifixion would come the resurrection and the ascension. He would receive his life back. Nevertheless, he had to first get through the next months. And they were way, way worse than anything I faced.

- When, if ever, have you been tempted to put a stop to your treatment?
- Provided you persevere, what will it mean to get your life back?
- What special meaning does 2 Corinthians 12:9 (see below) have for you?

Those months of radical chemotherapy definitely mark the worst period I have had to face in my life to date. Yet I praise God I made that tough decision and continued with my treatment.

In the nearly fifteen years since then, I have attended the weddings of both my sons and come to know my lovely daughters-in-law. I have witnessed my eldest granddaughter blossom from a toddler into a beautiful, vivacious young woman, and I have seen my first grandson race his way past puberty to manhood. I've held my third and fourth grandbabies in my arms and watched them develop into real little people. God really did give me back my life—and it's good.

**LET'S PRAY:** Lord God, it's so hard to deliberately go for treatment knowing it will make me ill. Help me to set my face toward the end of treatment, anticipating the beginning of a new way of life. Thank you for the miracle of modern medical techniques, Lord. Amen.

*But he said to me, "My grace is sufficient for you, for my power is made perfect in weakness." Therefore I will boast all the more gladly about my weaknesses, so that Christ's power may rest on me.*

2 CORINTHIANS 12:9

# 64

## Running a Marathon

READ: *Hebrews 12:1-3*

One morning I relaxed in front of the TV and watched coverage of the 89-kilometer* Comrade's Marathon. This oldest and largest ultramarathon in the world is run annually in South Africa between the inland city of Pietermaritzburg and the coastal city of Durban. One year the runners race uphill from Durban, and the alternate year they run down to the coast. The competitors train throughout the year, and only the fittest are able to compete. They learn to pace themselves and not overtax their bodies.

I watched as the occasional runner pulled out of the race. One had a cramp. Another had pushed himself too fast and couldn't continue. Yet another passed out from dehydration. These were all talented and trained athletes, yet they still had to take care of their bodies.

I thought about how chemotherapy attacked and destroyed all fast-growing cells. Cancer cells mutate at an alarming rate, and chemotherapy finds those cells and destroys them. However, white blood cells, which are necessary for the immune system, also develop fast. So chemo destroys them too. Fortunately the body quickly replaces the dead white cells, whereas the cancer cells are eliminated.

Suddenly I had a clearer picture of the battle taking place inside me. My blood vessels had to transport these damaged and dead cells until they could be eliminated from my body. No wonder I

*89 kilometers = 56 miles

had no energy. No wonder I felt drained and often was unable to think clearly. I now understood the need for extra rest. I had to consider my body and treat it with respect. It was doing the best it could under the circumstances. Pushing it beyond its limits would not help—it would only hinder my progress toward full health. I had to learn to pace myself, like the marathon runners.

In the first letter to the Corinthian church, Paul told believers he kept his body under control. I had to do the same.

- How can you help your body recover from treatment?
- What can you do to help your immune system get over each phase of treatment?
- In what ways do you take care of your body's increased nutritional needs?

No matter how well trained marathon runners may be, if they don't take care of their bodies and pace themselves carefully, they will run into trouble. The problem is, there's no training regimen for cancer treatment. We don't expect it, so we don't prepare for it. Once we're in the race, we need to do all we can to help our bodies cope with the extra stress. Like a race, cancer treatment doesn't last forever.

**LET'S PRAY:** Lord, sometimes it does feel as if I'm running a race. I become tired and need more rest. Help me to care for my body when it's assaulted by toxic drugs and treatment. Give me patience and perseverance to keep going. Thank you, Lord. Amen.

*I keep my body under control and make it my slave.*

1 CORINTHIANS 9:27 CEV

# 65

## Friends Who Count

READ: *3 John 1:1-6*

The apostle John was exiled to the small, rugged island of Patmos. Cut off from many of his friends and from his normal way of life, he learned to appreciate those who really cared.

I wasn't in exile, but during my time in the cancer valley I came to appreciate my true friends.

Some friends treated me as they had before my cancer diagnosis. They shared family news and told me about others in our congregation. They chatted about political issues and gave me their opinion about the latest TV news. I had no doubt of their prayerful support, and I could share openly how I felt.

On the other hand, some drained me of energy by their endless questions or negative attitudes.

The friends who truly helped were those who managed to look past the horror of a cancer diagnosis. Yes, they understood I was going through difficult treatment and at times really didn't feel up to chatting. I didn't feel threatened by a need to answer endless questions, nor did I feel I had to act a part and appear better than I really felt. They were there because they loved me, and when they left I always felt encouraged.

I didn't initially think of my oncologist as a "friend." After all, he was a medical professional who received payment to look after me. However, I soon came to appreciate his strong relationship with God. No matter what concerned me, I could always be assured of a listening ear, a sympathetic heart, and his caring prayers.

In addition to his medical expertise, he offered me spiritual support that I truly appreciated. I think there were times I nearly drove him to exhaustion with my endless questions as I grappled to understand what was happening to my body and second-guessed his every decision. Yet he always had time for me. He would reach for a book, open it to the appropriate place, and read passages out loud. Other times he drew diagrams for me on his trusty notepad.

Despite his busyness, he and many other friends were always there for me. I resolved that if the Lord restored me to full health, I would always have time for those in need. I planned to be the sort of friend that would bring encouragement and inspiration to those who wanted my company.

- Is there someone in your life who depletes your energy? How can you deal with this?
- Who cheers you up and makes you feel good?
- How can you show your appreciation, so that your supportive visitors will want to come and see you again?

Without friends, the cancer valley would be a lonely place indeed. One of the best things you can do for yourself is to encourage positive relationships. Try to be there for your friends when they need you, and appreciate the way they care for you.

**LET'S PRAY:** Father, thank you for friends. Thank you for people who love me when I'm not lovely. Help me to reflect more of your image and less of my own negative emotions. Amen.

*Give thanks to the God of heaven. His love endures forever.*

PSALM 136:26

# 66

## Snug as a Bird

**READ:** *Psalm 91:1-6*

It doesn't often snow in Johannesburg, but it does get bitterly cold. The houses don't have central heating, so by the early hours of the morning, bed is a good place to be. The winter during my cancer treatments, I could not get warm at night. Even curled up under our warm duvet and extra blankets, I still felt cold. I would snuggle against my husband and shiver, my teeth chattering as if I had a fever.

"We're going to get a feather duvet," my husband eventually announced after yet another sleepless night. "Even if we never use it again, we can't go on like this. You need your sleep." I suspected he wanted his too.

We went off to the shops and purchased an expensive duvet stuffed with duck down. I couldn't wait to try it out. Despite its bulkiness, I found it surprisingly light and cozy. As the night grew colder, the feathers trapped our body heat and kept us snug.

When I settled down to sleep that first night, I felt secure and comfortable. I remembered the words of the psalmist, "He will cover you with his feathers." I had often wondered about the meaning of that verse, but now I understood. I pictured a giant eagle spreading its mighty wings over its young, allowing them to hunker down and snuggle into warmth and comfort, unaware of the wind and the storm raging around them. I closed my eyes and sensed God's enormous wings spread over me. Nothing would be able to get by their protection. God was indeed my refuge.

- What area in your life most needs God's protective covering?
- What does Ruth 2:12 (see below) mean to you?
- How do you want to react when you read these words?

Getting a good night's sleep isn't the only time we need God as our refuge. Some folks need to nestle under God's protective wings with their marriage, their children, or some other relationship. Others need to crawl under his wings when their finances are out of control or when they need comfort from fear.

We don't always have to try to figure out a solution to our circumstances. Sometimes it is best to accept a situation as it stands and seek God's comfort and protection. Invite him to show you clearly if there's something you need to do about your problem. Meanwhile, enjoy the comfort of his presence.

**LET'S PRAY:** Lord God, thank you that even in the "shadow of death" you provide me with a place of comfort. You strengthen and equip me. You keep me company. Amen.

*May you be richly rewarded by the LORD, the God of Israel, under whose wings you have come to take refuge.*

RUTH 2:12

# 67

# Why Am I So Tired?

READ: *2 Thessalonians 3:3-5*

I let the book slide from my hands and onto the bedcover. How did she do it? The author had also gone through cancer treatment, yet she had continued to work part-time throughout the entire period. I felt like such a failure. It had been seven months since I last went to work.

Some mornings it took all my energy just to crawl out of bed, take a bath, get dressed, and put on makeup. I had never in my life napped during the daytime, yet now I slept most afternoons. I began to attend fabric painting classes one morning a week, when my white cell counts allowed me out of the house, and I enjoyed this new hobby. I made cards "from a secret friend" to send to children who had been removed from their families for safety reasons.

Whenever possible, I studied HTML code and put my lessons into practice developing a website with so many bells and whistles it would never get online. On some good days I went shopping with my husband or attended a church function. But most of the time I had to stay home. And I couldn't go to work.

I mentioned my frustration to a friend, who looked at me in amazement.

"Shirl, you're never idle," she encouraged. "You make the effort to look good. Even when you're resting, you keep yourself busy. Don't forget—your body is working harder than it ever has before."

She was right. Apart from my physical activities, my body never rested. Along with the cancer cells, the chemotherapy drugs destroyed many of my red blood cells, so there were less of them to carry oxygen around my body. While my body worked to destroy the unwanted cell debris, my bone marrow struggled to replace damaged white cells with new ones. My impaired immune system continued to fight threatened infections with its depleted resources. Even when I slept, my body worked on. No wonder I was exhausted.

If I'd had a desk job in an office, there would have been days when I could spend time at work. However, I had worked in a pathology laboratory. Now my colleagues didn't even allow me to walk in the door when I went to have blood drawn, because the risk of infection in the waiting room was too high. My husband had to call one of them to come and draw blood while I sat in the car.

My situation was different from the woman who wrote the book I was reading. I had to stop comparing myself with others and just be the best "me" I could be. God knew my body was working harder than ever before.

- Whom do you compare yourself to? Is it a fair comparison?
- How do you care for your body?
- What new hobby or interest can you try?

The Lord knows how much we are capable of and how much we achieve each day. If he is happy, then we shouldn't expect more of ourselves. The important thing is to encourage our bodies by allowing them time to recover.

LET'S PRAY: Lord, forgive me for being resentful over what I can't do instead of rejoicing in what I can. Thank you for the small pulses of energy I experience at times. Help me to use them wisely. Amen.

*I know your deeds . . . and that you are now doing more than you did at first.*

REVELATION 2:19

# 68

## Teach Me to Fly

READ: *Psalm 55:4-8*

Shortly before my cancer diagnosis, Rob and I had spent a day at a sanctuary for birds of prey. Set on a high hill surrounded by mountains and valleys, this fascinating center is dedicated to the conservation of indigenous raptors. We marveled at the size of some of these magnificent creatures, and we laughed at the "gobble and squabble" of the vulture feeding time. I loved our time in Eagle Alley where we saw the "big five" of African eagle species. But the highlight of the day for me was an hour-long presentation of some birds in flight.

I gazed in wonder at the handsome African fish eagle, with a wingspan of over six feet. This gigantic bird rose gracefully from its handler's arm and soared into the sky, higher and higher, then headed toward the distant mountains. It flew across the rugged valley and eventually disappeared from view. While the handler spoke to us, I wondered how she knew for sure the eagle would return.

Some minutes later, we spotted a speck in the distance. It drew closer until we were able to recognize the shape and flight of the returning bird. It rushed in at a tremendous speed and landed gently on the handler's arm.

During my treatment, I saw a photograph of an African Fish Eagle and remembered that wonderful day. "How I wish I could be like that eagle," I said to Rob. "To be able to soar effortlessly over the next few months . . . wouldn't it be wonderful?" If only I could fly into the heavens and look down on my cancer experience.

Then when the treatment came to an end, I could whoosh back from my lofty height and carry on with life. It sounded like an ideal plan to me.

I took another look at Isaiah 40:31. The King James Version puts it this way: "But they that wait upon the LORD shall renew their strength; they shall mount up with wings as eagles." Then I noticed something I'd missed before: God doesn't tell *us* to renew our strength or mount up with wings. He tells us to wait upon him, and when we do, we *will* renew our strength. All we have to do is learn to be patient. And that isn't easy.

- If God granted you wings, what part of your life would you like to soar above?
- What positive experiences or lessons might you miss if you were able to fly above the hard parts of life?
- Think of at least one thing of value you have learned in the cancer valley.

Much as I would have loved to be able to soar over the next months, in hindsight I can see all that I would have missed. My experiences in the cancer valley were tough. The lessons I learned were difficult. Yet I am grateful to God for them. I am a better person and a stronger Christian because of what I went through.

**LET'S PRAY:** Father God, thank you for the picture of an eagle. Thank you for your promise that if I wait on you, I *will* have my strength renewed. Help me, Lord, to wait on you. Help me to have patience. Amen.

*How priceless is your unfailing love, O God! People take refuge in the shadow of your wings.*

PSALM 36:7

# 69

## The Face in the Mirror

READ: *1 Peter 3:3-4*

One morning I got up and made my way to the bathroom. As I washed my hands, I happened to glance in the mirror—and froze in horror. Staring back at me was a woman I didn't recognize. Her face was devoid of color. She had no lips; the outline of her mouth blended with the surrounding skin. Her huge eyes were dark and sunken and stared back at me in equal horror. Her face was covered in brown spots.

On my way back to bed, I dragged a medical book from the shelf. I propped myself on pillows and paged through the book.

When my sons returned from church, they came through to my bedroom. A look of shock flashed across Stephen's face before he could hide it. "Hi," he said as he lowered himself to the floor by the side of my bed.

My youngest son, David, walked through the door. Alarm shot across his face. He sat down on the edge of my bed and glanced at the book on my lap. "What're you looking for, Mom?"

My eyes filled with tears. "I'm trying to figure out what's wrong. I can't find a disease with brown spots."

I felt both boys studying me. My heart beat faster. What if it was infectious? I should tell them to leave. But I needed them so badly.

Suddenly David burst out, "Hey! Those aren't spots! They're freckles! Don't you see? You've gone transparent, so they're standing out more than usual."

I stared at him in surprise, then my lips twitched as I realized he was right. Due to my extremely low cell count, my skin was so pale it had no color. Freckles that I normally disguised with makeup now stood out starkly against the "transparent" background. As the two boys burst out laughing, I didn't know whether to laugh or cry. So I did both. Tears of relief and weakness trickled down my cheeks as I chuckled at my silly panic.

"You'd better pass me my makeup," I said. "Maybe if I add some color I'll feel better."

- Does the face in your mirror sometimes give you a fright? Why not smile at the reflection, and maybe you'll both feel better.

- How do you dress? Try wearing cheerfully colored clothes.

- What does 1 Samuel 16:7 (below) mean to you?

Some days we look healthy. Other times our appearance can be alarming. We need to cultivate a realistic attitude toward the person in the mirror. After all, she's only an outward mask for the real person inside. As we do what we can to look good, we should then forget about the face in the mirror and develop an inner beauty that will shine through our transparent complexions.

LET'S PRAY: Lord, it's frightening when I look in the mirror and don't recognize my own reflection. Help me to remember that I'm still the same person. Remind me that you don't even look at my outward appearance; you love the "me" on the inside. Amen.

*The LORD does not look at the things people look at. People look at the outward appearance, but the LORD looks at the heart.*

1 SAMUEL 16:7

# 70

# Unlikely Messenger

READ: *Jonah 2:10-3:5*

Imagine the scene: here comes Jonah, squishing along the beach. He's covered in the stomach contents of a fish and smells of vomit. His skin and hair are bleached white from stomach acids. Seaweed drapes around his shoulders. This man has a message from God? You have to be joking! Yet amazingly, the people of Nineveh listen to this unlikely messenger. They repent and turn to God.

At the beginning of my cancer treatment, I prayed that I would continue to be a witness to others of God's love. But toward the end of the year my thinning hair looked and felt like straw. My complexion was so pale and spotted that my sons said I was "transparent." My eyes looked sunken because I had lost so much weight. I don't think I looked quite as bad as Jonah must have looked, but I didn't see how God could use me. Yet surprisingly, he did.

Many people listened to what I had to say. They saw God at work in my life and asked questions about my faith. The Lord opened doors for me to write about my experiences so that others would be encouraged.

- In what ways can you encourage the people with whom you're in contact?
- What positive differences has cancer made in your life?
- Who can you tell about God's love as you've experienced it?

Perhaps one of the lessons in Jonah's story is that it's not the messenger who makes the difference in people's lives; it's the message. Even when we feel diminished and inadequate, God can still use us to spread his message of love and forgiveness.

**LET'S PRAY:** Father, thank you that I can still share your love with others. Please give me the words, and help me remember that I am only the messenger. You are the message. Amen.

*That is why, for Christ's sake, I delight in weaknesses, in insults, in hardships, in persecutions, in difficulties. For when I am weak, then I am strong.*

2 Corinthians 12:10

# 71

## Sword at the Ready

**READ:** *Matthew 4:1-11*

When I felt well, Satan left me alone. He would wait until my blood count hit bottom or when I felt crippled with bone pain in the early hours of the morning, and then he would pounce.

"If you are really a Christian, you could command this pain to leave."

"If God really cared about you, he would prevent your blood count from going so low."

"What makes you think you'll survive? Do you know how many people die of cancer?"

On and on it would go. One day I read these words in Ephesians: "Accept . . . the word of God as the sword which the Spirit gives you" (Eph. 6:17 GNT).

When Jesus was in the wilderness he faced far worse trials than I did during cancer treatment. After he had fasted for forty days and was really hungry, Satan arrived. He knew the strategy of attacking when a person's defenses are down.

"If you are God's Son, order these stones to turn into bread," he said. However, Jesus knew where the temptation came from.

"The Scripture says, 'Human beings cannot live on bread alone, but need every word that God speaks,'" Jesus responded (Matt. 4:4 GNT). Satan followed with a second temptation, then a third. Each time Jesus countered him with words from Scripture.

Finally, Satan gave up.

The passage in Ephesians reminded me I too had a sword, a weapon I could use against Satan. I collected all our Bibles and put them in strategic places around the house. I put one in the bathroom and another in the kitchen. I placed one in the lounge and one next to the computer. I kept a flashlight next to my bedside so that in the early hours of the morning I could read a verse open on my bedside table. I stuck individual Bible verses onto mirrors and door jambs.

As I learned to use the sword of the Spirit when Satan attacked, I grew more skillful. Often I was victorious. The most difficult part was learning to recognize the enemy before he inflicted wounds. I tried to reach out and grab the Bible at the first sign of trouble.

- When are you especially vulnerable to negative thoughts?
- What can you do to fight back?
- How can you make better use of your spiritual sword?

I wish I could say it always worked, but it didn't. My quickness to fight back faltered at times, as did my dexterity with the sword. However, the more time I spent reading the Bible, the more my faith grew. The stronger my faith, the quicker the victory.

**LET'S PRAY:** Thank you, Lord, for giving me such a powerful weapon. Forgive me for failing to use it more often. I wish I didn't have to fight like this, but help me to become a mighty warrior for you. You've given me power over Satan. Now help me to use it. Amen.

*Take the helmet of salvation and the sword of the Spirit, which is the word of God.*

EPHESIANS 6:17

# 72

## Proud for the Right Reasons

READ: *2 Corinthians 12:5-10*

I longed to be strong. Surely as a child of God I should be able to show people how well I coped with all things—even cancer. I should be able to smile through my pain, laugh through my tiredness, and keep my emotions under control at all times. After all, my strength was in the Lord—or was it?

As I read about Paul's life, my sufferings appeared trivial. He was mobbed, jailed, and beaten. He went without sleep or food and endured three shipwrecks. Yet he said, "I am most happy, then, to be proud of my weaknesses, in order to feel the protection of Christ's power over me" (2 Cor. 12:9 GNT).

I saw nothing about my weakness, my tiredness, my pain, or my mood swings to make me proud. Then I realized people would only see me as strong if they knew how difficult it was for me. If I moved smoothly through the treatment, didn't feel or talk about my pain, and my moods remained stable at all times, they wouldn't see the miracles God was doing. When they knew I had pain despite my forced smile, or if they saw tears of depression mock my feeble attempt to crack a joke, then they marveled at the strength the Lord had given me. When they heard me say, "I'm too weak to tackle this," and later saw that I had persevered through the task, they praised God for my persistence.

Then I saw the truth in Paul's words. When I admitted my weakness, I could boast—not in my own abilities, but in the strength God gave me.

- What weaknesses do you have that you struggle to hide?
- Have you heard someone share their weaknesses and how God helped them?
- Did that build you up, or did you despise them?

As an independent, capable person, I hated the weakness that cancer brought upon me. Yet as I surrendered to God and trusted him to see me through, I learned to appreciate his strength as well as the love and support of those around me. Truly, my strength did come from on high.

**LET'S PRAY:** Lord God, thank you for showing me I am special in your sight. Thank you for each of the unique qualifications that make me who I am. Help me to use each of these parts of my identity to draw others closer to you. Amen.

*Instead, in everything we do we show that we are God's servants by patiently enduring troubles, hardships, and difficulties.*

2 CORINTHIANS 6:4 GNT

# 73

## Goodness and Love

READ: *Psalm 23:1-6*

I have often found that if I take a well-known passage of Scripture and study it in depth, I find some nugget of truth I haven't seen before. This was certainly true when I was undergoing treatment.

One day I turned to Psalm 23 and let myself dwell on the picture of the Lord as my shepherd. That made me a sheep. Yes, I could see the similarities, many of which I preferred not to dwell on. He *makes* me lie down. He *leads* me. He *restores* me. He *guides* me. Clearly the Lord was in charge. Just as well. I shuddered at the mess a sheep would make of things.

When I reached verse 4, I paused. "Even though I walk through the valley of the shadow of death . . ." I identified with that picture too. I often felt as if I was in the shadow of death. I read on. "Goodness and love will follow me . . ." (v. 6). Suddenly the words "will follow" seemed to stand out from the page.

If I went for a walk and my husband followed me, I wouldn't see him in front of me. I wouldn't even catch sight of him on either side. I would only see him if I looked back.

I stared out the window and thought over the past year. Yes, it had been tough. I thought of the surgery—and the comfort I had received from my little stuffed lion. I looked back at all the friends, the cards, and the gifts I'd received. I saw how people had blessed me with their love. As my thoughts drifted to my family, I praised the Lord for *his* goodness shown through them.

David, our youngest, had shown amazing compassion and a newly gained patience. Stephen, our other son, had revealed leadership abilities we hadn't seen before. Our daughter, Debbie, despite being halfway across the globe, had done all she could to encourage and hold me up in prayer. And of course, my husband, Rob, had been an incredible support.

I thought about my medical team. My surgeon didn't approve of my choice of oncologist, and my oncologist didn't know my surgeon. Hardly ideal. Yet in their own diverse ways, they gave me full support when I needed it most. As I looked back over this difficult time, I saw how God's goodness and love had indeed followed me all the way.

- What does it mean to you that God's goodness and love follow you?
- As you look back over the past weeks, what areas of goodness and love can you see that you hadn't noticed before?
- How can you thank God today for his goodness and love?

Sometimes we are so conscious of our present suffering that we don't think to look back. Yet if we do, we will see evidence of God's goodness and love. We can then journey on with the assurance that the same God who was with us in the past will still be with us in the future. One day you will be able to look back on this time and say, "Yes, Lord. Your love and your goodness surely did follow me."

**LET'S PRAY:** Lord God, thank you so much for all the good things you've done for me in the past. Thank you for your goodness and love. Please help me to be more aware of the things you've done for me—and the things others have done as well. Amen.

*Trust in the LORD with all your heart and lean not on your own understanding; in all your ways submit to him, and he will make your paths straight.*

PROVERBS 3:5–6

# 74

## Divine Roller Coaster

READ: *Mark 1:9-14*

Soon after treatment began, I recognized the so-called cancer roller coaster. Physically, my body seemed like the spinning disc on the end of a yo-yo string—up and down, up and down, then whirling out of control. High cell count—low cell count; rosy cheeks—ashen face. Some mornings I awoke bright and optimistic, but by afternoon I hit the doldrums. Spiritually, I could wake up full of faith, but just a few hours later I doubted whether God even remembered me. Up the peaks, down into the valleys. At times I felt so unstable, I wondered if the cancer had gone to my brain.

As I looked at the life of Jesus, I realized his whole time on earth was a roller coaster ride. John the Baptist baptized him in the River Jordan. The Holy Spirit came upon him in the form of a dove. He heard his Father in heaven say, "This is my beloved Son in whom I am well pleased." What a series of emotional highs.

Immediately after, Jesus was led by the Spirit into the wilderness. *The wilderness?* It would have been bad enough if he had wandered there on his own, but the Holy Spirit led him. What a blow. Wild animals prowled, and he was tempted by Satan himself—a run of lows.

Satan left him for a period. Then angels came and ministered to him. How good that must have felt. Jesus was back on a high, but not for long.

His cousin was arrested and then executed. This wasn't just any cousin; John was God's advertising campaign for Jesus's ministry.

And now he was dead. How could God let that happen? Down. Way down. Jesus's peaks were far higher than anything I ever experienced. His valley experiences were far lower. Yet through it all he remained stable. Up and down—still, he continued to rely on God. He didn't allow his emotions to destroy his composure; no yo-yo behavior for the Son of God.

- How does it make you feel to know that Jesus himself experienced such roller coaster situations?
- What is the highest peak you can identify since your diagnosis?
- Can you identify specific times when you plunged down emotionally?

It's difficult to recognize the emotional roller coaster when you're on it. I found that being able to identify those times when I hit a low patch helped me deal with my feelings. I knew I would feel better shortly. At the same time, I found it difficult when members of the family tried to tell me I would feel better. To me it felt as if they didn't understand me. Of course, they didn't—but then neither did I.

**LET'S PRAY:** Lord God, sometimes it's difficult to deal with my emotions. Remind me often that, no matter if I'm on a high or in the depths of despair, nothing will ever separate me from your love. Thank you for that assurance. Amen.

*Neither height nor depth, nor anything else in all creation, will be able to separate us from the love of God that is in Christ Jesus our Lord.*

ROMANS 8:39

# 75

# The Unappreciated Gift

READ: *Matthew 8:1-4*

Jesus had just finished preaching the longest sermon recorded in Scripture, which today we know as the Sermon on the Mount. As he walked down the slopes of the mountain where he'd sat to teach, a large crowd followed him. Suddenly, a man knelt before him. The man was a leper, and he had no right to be near crowds of people. In fact, I wonder how he got so close to Jesus without people chasing him away. Jesus didn't send him away though. Instead, he reached out and touched him. *He touched a leper!* Immediately the leprosy left the man.

How thrilled that man must have been. His family and loved ones must have been ecstatic to have him home with them once more. But there would have been a downside to his healing. You see, leprosy causes a deterioration of pain receptors, which explains the horrific injuries suffered by those afflicted with the disease. Because they can't feel pain, lepers do not realize it when sores develop or they are injured. Once the man was healed, his feet would have become aware of the rough pebbles on the road. If he bumped his elbow, pain would have shot up his arm. If he touched a hot coal on the fire, he would have felt the burn. This man suddenly experienced pain—and he probably rejoiced.

My natural reaction to pain was definitely not one of rejoicing. As my wounds healed and my body worked overtime to replace the cells destroyed by radiation and chemotherapy, I often experienced pain. I complained to the Lord and anyone else who hadn't been quick enough to escape. After I read about the leper, I realized that pain was actually a gift—but it was still one I didn't appreciate.

- What pain or unpleasant side effects do you experience on a regular basis?
- In what ways are these a good sign?
- Try to think of one side effect you can praise the Lord for, even if it is a source of discomfort.

While it is difficult to appreciate pain, it often has a good side. Pain may show that the drugs are acting or that healing is taking place. The same applies to hair loss, nausea, and vomiting. Unpleasant though these and many other side effects are, they do encourage us that the treatment is at work in our bodies.

**LET'S PRAY:** Lord God, I can see that much of the pain and suffering I go through at the moment is a good sign, but it's still so hard to bear. Help me to praise you for the discomfort, and show me how best to handle it. Thank you, Lord. Amen.

*Why, my soul, are you downcast? Why so disturbed within me? Put your hope in God, for I will yet praise him, my Savior and my God.*

PSALM 42:11

# 76

# What Do You Mean, "It's Over"?

READ: *John 20:19-22*

We are all so different. Often we don't react to good news the way others would anticipate. The disciples were no exception. When Jesus rose from the dead, I would have expected them to celebrate with great excitement, wouldn't you? Instead, they cowered behind locked doors, terrified of the Jewish leaders.

I also had a strange reaction to what others saw as good news. For over a year I had been doing battle with cancer. I couldn't wait for the end of my treatment, when life would return to normal.

On November 16, 1998, one year and six days after my surgery for cancer, I arrived at the oncologist's office for my second-to-last chemotherapy. At last, the end was in sight. As I watched the yellow liquid run into the port in my chest, the oncologist smiled at me. "So, this is your last chemo."

"I wish," I said. "But I have one more to go."

He shook his head. "No, you've had enough. Your body needs a break. Your treatment's over."

I looked at him in alarm. My mind went in a whirl. He couldn't do this to me. I was supposed to have another one. I had tolerated this last regimen well. There was no reason to stop now.

"Are you sure?" I stammered. "I really don't mind having one more."

"You don't need it," he replied.

I felt bereft, badly treated, let down. He'd given up on me. Tears burned at the back of my eyes.

I often anticipated the joy I would feel when my treatment came to an end. Instead my heart pounded, my mouth felt dry, and I felt a ball of panic in my gut.

On the drive home, I struggled to understand my strange reaction. Why did I feel let down? I made a deliberate effort to sound excited as I phoned my family and the friends who had supported me through the difficult year.

When they commented, "You must be so thrilled!" I responded with, "I'm praising the Lord."

My mouth praised God; my emotions didn't.

As the day progressed, however, a curious shift occurred. I continued to praise, and soon I began to believe the news was good. By bedtime I could honestly say, "Thank you, Lord, that you've brought me to the end of this treatment. My future is in your hands."

- Are you excited or apprehensive about the time when your treatment will end?
- What plans do you have for life after treatment?
- Is there a situation in your life today where you can give thanks—even though you may not feel thankful yet?

Many cancer survivors experience the same emotions I did, especially if the length of treatment is cut short. In one sense, chemotherapy was proof of my fight against cancer. Suddenly I felt as if I'd quit fighting, but of course I hadn't. Chemotherapy was only one tool in my arsenal. My body would continue the fight—and God would still be in control.

**LET'S PRAY:** Loving Father God, you help me so much, yet at times I rely on treatment and doctors. Help me to always remember that they are simply tools in your hand. Amen.

*Let the weak say, I am strong.*

JOEL 3:10 KJV

# 77

## Starting Over

READ: *Ruth 1:22-2:3*

Naomi was an Israelite who lived for ten years in the land of Moab, a country God referred to as his "washbasin" in Psalm 60:8. It was not a good place for God's children to be. Since Naomi had left her home country of Judah, her husband and both her sons had died, leaving her and her two daughters-in-law widowed.

Sometime after the third family death, Naomi pulled herself together and decided to return to her own country. One of her daughters-in-law, Ruth, went with her. Bethlehem, Naomi's hometown, was more than thirty miles from Moab—a long and dangerous journey for two vulnerable women. There were no coaches or trains, no rest stops or motels along the way. It couldn't have been an easy decision for Naomi, but her mind was made up. I can imagine her thinking, "This can't go on. There must be more to life."

The dry and dusty terrain made walking hard, and it would have taken the women over a week to complete the distance. When they arrived in Bethlehem, they faced all sorts of difficulties. Yet while they wondered where their next meal would come from, God was putting together an exciting future for them both. Little did Naomi know when she made the difficult decision to start over that God was offering Ruth and her a new beginning. God was planning a wedding and a baby—a baby who would one day be grandfather to the great King David.

Within a year of the end of my cancer treatment, Rob and I moved home to the other side of South Africa, and I too made a life-changing decision. I longed to get back to work, but there were no opportunities for nursing in my new location. Besides, I still lacked the stamina to cope with long hours and demanding work. For a while I battled with my new way of life. In fact, I hated it. Why had God brought me through the tough time with cancer? Surely he had better plans for me than having to sit at home looking for ways to fill my time.

And of course, he did. Like Naomi, I had to accept that my life had changed. It would never be the same. "This can't go on," I decided. "There must be more to life." Once I reached that point and surrendered my own plans to God, I found he had an exciting future planned for me—a future that so far has involved two transatlantic flights to America and a new career as a published author.

- What part of your life may never be the same again?
- Have you surrendered it to the Lord, trusting him with your future?
- Can you imagine what he may have in store for you? Don't worry if you can't. That makes it all the more exciting.

Naomi had to move from Moab. I had to give up my dreams of returning to hospital nursing. God has exciting plans for your future too. Are you perhaps preventing them from happening because you want to hang on to your past way of life? Maybe it's time to surrender your ideas and ask God to show you his. And do you know what? They'll be much better than yours.

**LET'S PRAY:** Lord God, I can't go on like this. I'm sure you have more planned for my life. Please show me, and guide me in your way. Thank you so much. Amen.

*Those who sow with tears will reap with songs of joy.*

PSALM 126:5

# 78

## Angels Unaware

READ: *Matthew 28:1-10*

Joseph of Arimathea placed the body of Jesus in his own tomb. He rolled a massive boulder across the entrance. Roman soldiers sealed the tomb and then placed men on guard duty. No one could get in, and certainly no one could get out. Then God sent an angel who rolled away the stone.

I used to think the heavenly messenger rolled away the stone to allow Jesus out. Then one day I understood that Jesus was no longer there when the angel arrived. He had already risen from the dead. God opened the tomb to show those outside that he was at work.

During my twelve months of radical and life-threatening treatment for cancer, I often felt trapped inside my body. Then God would send someone to "roll away the stone" and show me he was at work in my life.

One day, when our finances had reached a critical stage, we found an envelope containing a large amount of money stuffed under the front door. On another occasion, after my treatment had been canceled due to a dangerously low blood count, a family member gave us a week's vacation at a luxury resort. Flowers, cards, and unexpected gifts assured me that many people loved me and were praying for me.

These were not medical essentials. They didn't open the way to a cancer cure. Rather, they opened my eyes to see God at work. I thank God for his human messengers who helped me see past death and suffering. He sent them exactly when I needed them.

- When, if ever, did you see God at work in your life through another person?
- In what ways do you need to see God at work in your life? Ask him now to show you where he's at work.
- What will you thank God for today?

When we are in pain or feel as if we'll never again be able to keep food down, it is easy to take for granted the things people do to help us. Sometimes the simple act of saying "thank you" helps us to move past the situation and see a glimmer of light at the end of the tunnel—or from an empty tomb.

**LET'S PRAY:** Loving Father, thank you that even when I feel trapped in my situation, you are still at work. Help me to recognize your messengers and say "thank you." Amen.

*For this very reason, Christ died and returned to life so that he might be the Lord of both the dead and the living.*

ROMANS 14:9

# 79

## A Lesson from Nature

READ: *Philippians 3:10-16*

Soon after my final treatment, I sat on a bench in a small park. At my feet, multitudes of black ants scurried around in seeming chaos. One tiny ant, burdened by a dead insect at least ten times its size, raced from the pack. It weaved around weeds, under roots, and over tufts of grass. No matter what stood in its way, it kept moving forward. I watched in fascination and tried to see where it was headed.

A sudden gust of wind blew, and the little insect somersaulted backward. I watched as it turned itself around to its original position and adjusted its load. Seconds later, it resumed its journey, speeding along at the same busy pace. After several minutes and many setbacks, it reached a tiny hole and disappeared from view. I marveled at how it had persevered until it reached its nest.

I compared myself to that little ant. The goal of total health seemed so far away. At times I couldn't even imagine having my health and strength back. It seemed that every time I took a few steps forward, a wind came along and blew me backward. Some mornings I felt strong, but by afternoon I needed to crawl onto my bed and sleep.

There were days I tackled small tasks around the house with enthusiasm. Halfway through, however, I would have to stop as it became too much for me. Sometimes it seemed easier to say, "This is too hard. Maybe I won't even try."

I wondered if this was what King Solomon referred to when he said, "Learn a lesson from the ant." That tiny insect, which I would never see again, taught me a valuable lesson: pick yourself up, redistribute your burden, and take the next steps forward. Sometimes it would be too much and I'd stumble back. But I needed to learn to renew my strength and start forward once more.

- At what times, or in what situations, do you feel like giving up?
- Is there a task you want to tackle but you're not sure you can cope?
- How can you break that task into tiny steps to make it more manageable?

When faced with a task that would have been easy in pre-cancer days, it's often wise to sit down and draw up a plan. Divide it into small, doable steps and tackle one at a time. Even if it takes a week to complete, at least you're moving forward. Eventually it will get done—if you persevere.

**LET'S PRAY:** Lord God, thank you that you will never give me a burden to carry that is beyond my ability. Please help me to persevere and not give up. Amen.

*Look at an ant. Watch it closely; let it teach you a thing or two.*

PROVERBS 6:6 MESSAGE

# 80

## Tiny Steps

READ: *Psalm 84:5-12*

My year of treatment was behind me, yet even a short stroll required regular breaks. I could only manage a few minutes at the shops before stopping to rest. How I longed for the days when I bubbled with vitality. "I wish I could get my strength back," I would complain, but the days passed and my energy remained on a plateau. One day I decided to stop wishing and do something about it.

Knowing I couldn't walk far, I set myself a tiny goal. I walked slowly out my front gate, around the corner, and back in the other gate. It took me two minutes, and I was tired but determined. I had taken the first steps on my journey back to strength. The next day I walked past the second gate before turning back. The walk took three minutes. Each day I pushed for a few more steps, one more minute. The farther I walked, the more encouraged I felt. The better I felt about my progress, the farther I walked. My energy crept back and my coping skills returned.

In the Old Testament, David made a similar observation. After he'd watched the people's pilgrimage toward the temple, he said, "They grow stronger as they go" (Ps. 84:7 GNT). As long as I sat and thought about the challenge before me, I didn't make progress. I had to trust God for the strength and ability, then take those first steps for myself.

- In what situation do you feel frustrated by your lack of progress?
- What plan can you make to move forward, albeit with tiny steps?
- How will you encourage yourself when you see improvement?

Sometimes we forget what a traumatic ordeal our bodies have been through. We need to be patient and set tiny goals. Then we will see our progress and be encouraged.

**LET'S PRAY:** Father, you know the longing of my heart. Show me where to start, and then please help me take the first step. Amen.

*If you do what the LORD wants, he will make certain each step you take is sure.*

PSALM 37:23 CEV

# 81

## Live in the Now

READ: *Luke 4:28-32*


Though my treatment was finished, for the next five years I faced frequent tests and visits to my oncologist. Eventually they would reduce in number until they were only once a year. Forever. I would never be able to wipe cancer from my history.

Dr. Phil, the well-known television host, says in his book *Life Strategies: Stop Making Excuses! Do What Works, Do What Matters*: "The value of history lies in making you aware that someone has placed a filter over your eyes and mind that influences the way you see the world." He's right. Cancer places a filter over our eyes and minds. He continues, "The only thing worse than the event itself would be allowing that event to destroy that person's entire life by coloring how they see the world thirty, forty, or fifty years later."*

I heard of a woman who became a cancer survivor. She spent the rest of her life dreading a return of the disease. Every symptom that appeared, she suspected the worst. She lived for another thirty-five years and died of a heart attack in her nineties. Those spoiled hours of worry robbed her of so much joy—all for nothing.

A crowd once wanted to throw Jesus over a cliff, but Jesus knew his time had not yet come. So he walked away from the experience and continued to live to the full. He never lost sight of his mission here on earth. He knew that one day he would give his life as a

---

*Phillip C. McGraw, *Life Strategies: Doing What Works, Doing What Matters* (New York: Hyperion, 2000), 146.

sacrifice for mankind—but that was in the future. For his life to make a difference, he had to live in the present.

I resolved to leave the future up to God. Yes, I would have my tests. Yes, I would do all I could to avoid a repeat of cancer. Yes, I would pray it would never return. But I would not allow it to rob me of the present. I could never wipe cancer from my history, but it didn't need to rule how I lived each day.

- What causes you to panic about a possible recurrence of cancer?
- Which verse of Scripture would be helpful to use as a sword when these thoughts come? (See "Sword at the Ready," p. 154.)
- In what ways can you relegate cancer to your *history* and anticipate a healthy future?

Cancer is fifteen years behind me. I still live my life with caution. I have an annual checkup that involves fewer tests than before. I take care of my health and remain vigilant, but life in the now is good. Cancer doesn't rule my life.

**LET'S PRAY:** Loving Father, I admit I'm often afraid of the future. I don't think I could face having to go through this again. I know I will never forget my history with cancer, nor should I. But please help me to live the present to the full and leave my future in your hands. Amen.

*Cast all your anxiety on him because he cares for you.*

1 PETER 5:7

# 82

## Who Am I?

READ: *Mark 8:27-29*

A few months after my treatment ended, I went to my general practitioner about a non-cancer issue. After checking me, he ordered X-rays. Then he said words that caused me to bristle.

"Seeing you're a cancer patient, we need to exclude . . ."

"I'm *not* a cancer patient," I interrupted. "I *had* cancer. It's been removed and my body treated for any possible spread. I'm a cancer survivor. Please don't call me a cancer patient again."

He gave a slight smile and inclined his head. "Just as you like. I still think we need to exclude . . ."

That was fine, and I agreed with him. But I resolved never to accept the title "cancer patient" again. Not unless, God forbid, it put in another appearance.

So, who am I?

I'm a pastor's wife. I'm mother to three adult children and mother-in-law to their three spouses. I'm grandmother to four of the world's greatest kids. I'm an RN and a writer. I'm a child of God. And I'm a cancer survivor.

Each of those descriptions adds to who I am. Each carries a set of responsibilities—and that includes the term *cancer survivor*. It's part of my identity.

Jesus never had an identity crisis. He knew who he was, and he knew why he had come to earth.

"I am the bread of life" (John 6:35). "I am the way, the truth and the life" (John 14:6). "I am the good shepherd" (John 10:14). And there are more such statements.

One day he asked his disciples, "Who do people say I am?" They gave several replies. Then Jesus became personal: "But who do *you* say I am?"

- Who are you? List the identities that make you *you*.
- Did you include "cancer survivor"? If your answer is no, why not?
- If Jesus asked you today, "Who do you say I am?" how would you answer?

Early in my treatment I read a book that described a survivor as someone who is still alive after the event. Think about it: after a tornado or tsunami or landslide, emergency services rush to find survivors. No matter how badly the person may be injured, he or she has survived the initial crisis and is therefore a survivor. The same is true of someone who's had surgery or any other treatment for cancer. The moment you come around from that anesthetic, you are a survivor.

So who are you? Included in your list of identities should be the statement, "I am a cancer survivor." No matter how you feel, no matter your prognosis—you are a survivor. Keep reminding yourself of this.

**LET'S PRAY:** Thank you, Lord, for all the qualities and attributes that come together to make me "me." Thank you that you created me and that you know me completely, inside and out. Thank you that right now, regardless of how I feel or what my prognosis may be, I am a survivor. Amen.

*Therefore, if anyone is in Christ, the new creation has come: the old has gone, the new is here!*

2 CORINTHIANS 5:17

# 83

## Absolute Guarantee

READ: *John 14:1–3*

On my first postoperative visit to the surgeon he had said, "With the right chemotherapy, there's a good chance you could live another five years." I didn't want five years. I wanted to live to an old age. There was no such guarantee.

When I first received a diagnosis of breast cancer, friends told me after five years I would be pronounced "clean." However, as I read about the subject, I soon learned there is never a guarantee it won't return.

Yet when I read the book of Revelation, I read about something far better than five years, and it comes with a guarantee. One day I will reach a place in my life where there will be no death—ever. My life here on earth is transitory, and that has nothing to do with cancer. From the moment of my conception, it was preordained that one day I would die.

Although I had attended church since early childhood, I was nearly nineteen when I realized I could have a personal relationship with Jesus Christ. From then on, I knew what it meant to belong to God. I had the assurance of a home in heaven after death. There will be no suffering, no crying, no pain . . . and no cancer.

- When, if ever, did you make a definite commitment to Jesus Christ?*

*If you've never committed your life to Christ, please read "New Relationship" on p. 192.

- What steps can *you* take to help you reach old age here on earth?
- What appeals to you most about life in heaven?

I still want to reach my senior years here on earth, but how good to know that, although very little on this earth is definite, my well-being in eternity is absolutely guaranteed.

**LET'S PRAY:** Lord Jesus, thank you that my place in heaven is guaranteed through your death on the cross. Please give me the assurance that you've forgiven my sins, so one day I will live with you in eternity. Thank you, Lord. Amen.

*He will wipe every tear from their eyes. There will be no more death or mourning or crying or pain.*

REVELATION 21:4

# 84

## New Life

READ: *Isaiah 35:1-4*

I had struggled through droughts of low immunity, pain, fear, and uncertainty, and I had made it. My final chemo was behind me. My blood tests looked good. Yet I still had no energy. One day I would think I was getting back to health, the next I'd be exhausted and nervous. Every little lump or ache caused a tightening in my throat: *Is it back?*

One day I remembered a car trip we had taken across the South African Karoo Desert. We drove along parched roads and crossed miles of desolate land where a few tufts of brown grass struggled for existence. Sporadic thorn trees offered little shade. Heat shimmered over the vastness. It didn't seem possible the region would ever see life again.

Yet I knew that despite appearances, the spring rains would soon come. Although this part of the desert would only receive a few inches of rain in the year, it would be enough. Beautiful, exotic wildflowers would spring up overnight. The stark area would transform into the sea of color for which it is famous. Indeed, the desert would "burst into bloom" (Isa. 35:2).

I reminded myself that the same Creator God who watched over this barren land and knew exactly when and where to send the rains also watched over me. Yes, there would be life again. My energy would return. My emotional desert would bloom once more. I just had to be patient.

- How does your fear of a possible recurrence prevent you from enjoying your life right now?
- When did you last smell a rose or admire a snowdrop?
- Where can you go to enjoy time in a garden, to remind yourself of God's care over creation? If you're not able to go out, perhaps ask someone to find pictures for you.

I live in Africa where droughts are common. Perhaps where you live floods are more common. Or perhaps you have to contend with heavy snowfalls. Wherever you are, there is likely a time in your year when flowers are less bountiful. Yet God knows exactly what is needed to bring them to full bloom at the appointed time. And he knows just what we need to bring us through this difficult time in the rugged cancer valley.

**LET'S PRAY:** Lord God, as I look at flowers I thank you for the beauty of your world. Thank you for bringing me through my treatment. Help me to trust you with my future. Amen.

*Consider how the wild flowers grow. They do not labor or spin. Yet I tell you, not even Solomon in all his splendor was dressed like one of these.*

LUKE 12:27

# 85

# A Living Tapestry

READ: *Isaiah 55:9-13*

S ome years after my treatment ended, my husband and I visited Stirling Castle in Scotland. Scaffolding supported some walls, and many craftsmen were hard at work to restore the ancient site to its former beauty.

In a special workroom, teams of three weavers at a time labored together on an immense tapestry. They sat in a row in front of a huge standing loom. The weavers could only see the tiny areas in front of them. They followed a printed template and could only work with the colors illustrated on the canvas background.

It didn't seem possible that the riot of colors and tangled threads could possibly fit into a logical design. On the wall, a full-scale detailed print showed the magnificent picture the tapestry would eventually become. As I studied the print, I tried to imagine it without blacks or grays. If the scene comprised only interesting colors, it would be like a kaleidoscope—broken shapes of colors with no sense.

The tapestry would take three years to finish. When the weavers completed their tasks, the entire canvas would be unrolled. At last they would see the results of their years of labor. The finished masterpiece would then hang in the castle for visitors to view.

My life during treatment often resembled that tapestry on the loom. I could only see the piece in front of me, with its crossed and tangled threads and ugly knots, and I often felt discouraged and confused. The cancer diagnosis didn't fit into my plans for the future at all. The dark side effects and miserable times lacked interest or color and showed no signs of beauty. Day after day I trudged through the rigors of treatment, wondering how it would turn out in the end. Could God really turn this into something beautiful? It seemed impossible.

Yet God could see the full picture. He knew the great plan for my life even before my birth. He knew my life needed a touch of black here, a dash of uninteresting color there, to make sense of the design. One day he will unroll the canvas and I'll see the result of my years here on earth. Then I will understand and appreciate the times of darkness.

- What dark threads are in your life's tapestry today?
- Which tangles and knots in your life can be made beautiful only through divine intervention?
- When you see the finished picture of your life, what will be the first part you want to look at?

Dark colors are essential to any tapestry or painting. Without them, there would be no picture. A frame that contains no color is simply a black shape. Our lives are not black shapes, nor are they kaleidoscopes. They are beautiful, orderly designs meant to show God's glory. No matter how black things appear right now, the light and dark shades will eventually blend together. Take heart. Brighter colors are coming.

**LET'S PRAY:** Thank you, Lord, that there's a reason for times of dark as well as of gaiety and beauty. Help me to concentrate on the now and trust you with the final outcome. Amen.

*Before I formed you in the womb I knew you, before you were born I set you apart.*

JEREMIAH 1:5

# 86

## Beware of the Little Foxes

READ: *Proverbs 30:24-28*

Before my husband and I were married, we often climbed the famous Table Mountain in Cape Town. One day we decided to take a new route. After a few hours Rob called a halt.

"We're on the wrong side of the gorge," he said. "We should be across there." He pointed to the other side of a deep ravine.

I couldn't see any reason to be concerned. "So what? As long as we're climbing, we must surely end up at the top?"

After a few minutes' deliberation, we decided to press on. After all, why turn around and go back for what could be a considerable distance, just to get on the other side?

Several hours later, after scrambling with difficulty over a section of sheer rock, we recognized our mistake. The way ahead was not safe for amateur climbers, but we couldn't turn back. We had no ropes. Had we attempted to get back down the cliff we had just scrambled up, we would almost certainly have slipped and fallen, probably to our death. We had no option but to persevere. After a number of scares, we eventually reached the top as night was falling. We still had to figure out how to get back down the mountain. The earlier decision to keep going on the wrong side of the gorge was a small decision—but it nearly cost us our lives.

It's a pity we hadn't learned a lesson from Solomon. In Song of Songs he warns us that if the little foxes are not caught, they will bring ruin to the vineyard (2:15). In the same way, little choices, if they are wrong, may ruin our lives. We think we can sort them out later. But, as we found out on that mountainside, when little mistakes are not rectified they can develop into big problems. As soon as we recognize we've veered from the correct path, we need to stop and ask God how to get back on track.

People often ask me what caused my cancer. I have no idea. Perhaps there were little decisions along the way where I made a wrong move. Maybe they didn't seem important at the time. My decision to listen to my gynecologist, who didn't support regular mammograms, nearly cost me my life. Praise God I finally insisted on one, but I almost waited too long. I realized that I needed to take better care of my health. I had to make wiser decisions and watch my lifestyle.

- What little decisions or responses can you think of that have helped you in your cancer journey?
- Is there an area in your life now where you're allowing "little foxes" to run riot?
- Can you think of one habit you need to drop or alter in your life?

It's easy to become so wrapped up in our discomfort, pain, and weakness that we don't notice the little foxes at work. Yet sometimes we need to make changes, even small ones. If we take care of the little things, we will find the bigger issues easier to handle.

**LET'S PRAY:** Father, help me to see the importance of little things. Forgive me for the times I press on even when I realize I'm not heading where you want me to be. Give me the strength to make changes where necessary and take better care of my body. Amen.

*Catch for us the foxes, the little foxes that ruin the vineyards, our vineyards that are in bloom.*

SONG OF SONGS 2:15

# 87

## New Values

READ: *2 Corinthians 11:24-30*

According to Hebrews 12:28, God's kingdom cannot be shaken, but that is certainly not true of our lives. Look at the apostle Paul. He faced floggings, was shipwrecked three times, and was lost at sea. He faced hunger, thirst, and countless dangers. Many of his previously held convictions were shaken, and he found himself with a new set of values. Yet he continued to serve the Lord and his church. The many hazards he survived made him a stronger and more effective teacher of the gospel.

Cancer shook my life with a series of upheavals and emotional quakes. At times my own convictions seemed uncertain. Did God really care? I believed he did, but why then did he allow me to feel so dreadfully ill? Did he still heal today? I knew he did, yet suddenly doubts crept in and made me wonder. My belief system and even my personality seemed to be under fire. How would this struggle with cancer affect me? Would I be the same person as I was when I was diagnosed?

Then one day I received inspiration from nature. A friend gave me a beautiful arrangement of proteas. These spectacular flowering plants, indigenous to South Africa, have amazing built-in survival systems. In some varieties, the seeds are protected in small cones sealed by a resin. When wild bush fires sweep over the plants, the resin melts and the seeds are carried away by the updraft from the fire.

Central to my floral arrangement was a King Protea, the national flower of South Africa. The flower heads of these magnificent plants can be up to twelve inches in diameter. They occur in several different colors and over eighty varieties. Fire causes the King Protea to send out new shoots from buds growing deep in its underground stem.

Tourists travel from all over the world to marvel at the Cape Floral Kingdom, an area especially famous for its annual display of proteas. Yet without the intense heat of fire, these magnificent plants would never reach their potential, and indeed some varieties would die out completely.

I wondered what the heat of cancer would do in my life. I couldn't wait for the fire to be over, and I looked forward to what God would produce in me.

- How is your life being shaken at the moment?
- Which preconceptions do you need to let go of?
- What, if any, important values are peeking through the ashes of your old life?

When life is going according to plan, we don't stop to question our daily habits. When a crisis erupts we find ourselves unable to cope with everything we want to do. Maybe it's time to sift through our lives and see if there are things we should stop so that our faith and abilities can be free to grow. Maybe there are new values we need to embrace. No, we won't be the same when this is over, but like those proteas, perhaps we will be able to reach our true potential.

**LET'S PRAY:** Lord, please protect my faith in the flames of the cancer fire. One day, please, may I look around and see a new season of beauty around me? Thank you. Amen.

*Therefore, since we are receiving a kingdom that cannot be shaken, let us be thankful, and so worship God acceptably with reverence and awe.*

HEBREWS 12:28

# 88

## A Time to Be Patient

READ: *Mark 14:29–31, 72*

Jesus warned the disciples that people would ridicule him and ultimately put him to death. He also said they would desert him. Peter became indignant and assured Jesus that even if the others ran away, he never would.

A few days later, Jesus's warnings came true. He was arrested and mocked, and the disciples fled. Peter denied even knowing Jesus. He had overestimated his own strength and courage.

In the early stages of recovery, I often overrated my strength too.

One morning I awoke feeling cheerful. I decided to go to the shops on my own and get the few items we needed.

When I said good-bye to Rob with the car keys in my hand, he hesitated. "Are you sure you're up to this?"

I bristled. "Rob, it's a three-minute drive to the shops. I'll get what we need and be home in no time." The sun beamed down on me, reinforcing my feeling of confidence. I relished the sense of being in control of my life once more.

At the grocery store, I took a shopping cart and started to select items from the shelves. All went well for about five items. Then without warning, the shelves spun out of focus. My knees wobbled and I had to hang on to the cart handle for support. After a short period everything drifted back into focus, but I knew I couldn't go on. Shaken, I parked my shopping cart alongside the shelves and made my way back to the car. I sat there for a few minutes. Tears of weakness and disappointment trickled down my cheeks. I prayed for help, then drove slowly home, hugging the curb.

I dropped into the chair in Rob's office. "I couldn't do it," I said miserably. "I had to leave the cart parked in the aisle, right in the middle of the shop. What's the matter with me?"

Rob got to his feet and held me tight. "What's the matter with you? You've just ended treatment for cancer, that's what's the matter. The drugs are still in your system, Shirl. Don't push yourself. Give yourself time."

My patient husband settled me in the lounge with a cup of tea and then drove to the shop to find my cart of groceries and complete the shopping.

- When, if ever, have you pushed yourself beyond your endurance?
- How long has it been since you finished treatment? Are you expecting too much too soon?
- Won't it be wonderful to feel well again? Is there something practical you can do to build up your strength?

During treatment, I learned to accept my body's limitations. But when chemotherapy ended, I forgot the drugs were still in my system. It took months before the drug-related symptoms eased and even longer before my strength returned. I wish someone had explained this to me in advance.

**LET'S PRAY:** Lord, thank you that the treatment is over. I want to return to my full strength as soon as possible. Please give me patience. Amen.

*Then Jesus said, "Let's go to a place where we can be alone and get some rest."*

MARK 6:31 CEV

# 89

## Something Good? You're Kidding

READ: *2 Kings 5:1-15*

When I faced the diagnosis of cancer, many people said to me, "I don't understand why you have to go through this." Neither did I.

Years later I can tell of many good things that came out of my cancer battle. My life story changed, no question, but in many ways for the better. God took the bad experience of cancer and turned it into something good.

In the Bible we read how Naaman, the brave commander of the Syrian army, had a similar experience. He suffered from the terrifying disease of leprosy.

One day, a little maid came to Naaman's wife with news of a prophet in her home country of Israel. She believed he could cure Naaman of his leprosy. A few days later, the afflicted officer and his entourage set off to visit Elisha.

Naaman anticipated an interview with the great prophet. Instead, Elisha sent a servant to answer the door.

Naaman probably expected the holy man would pray to his god and the leprosy would be cured. "Go to the Jordan River and wash in it seven times," Elisha instructed through his servant.

Naaman turned his chariots around and left in anger.

"Why couldn't the prophet come out and talk to me?" he fumed. "What's wrong with our rivers in Damascus? They're as good as any of the rivers in Israel."

His servants persuaded him to give the Jordan a try. Naaman walked down to the banks of the river. He waded into the water and bathed once, twice . . . seven times, as Elisha had told him. After the seventh time, to his amazement and delight, his skin appeared as smooth as a child's. The leprosy had disappeared.

Naaman progressed from his problem to God's solution, which involved more than physical healing. He came to know the true God, something that would never have happened if he hadn't had leprosy.

- What blessing can you see so far that has come out of your sojourn in the cancer valley?
- How does your post-treatment lifestyle differ from your pre-cancer days?
- Where have you grown in your spiritual life as a result of your battle with cancer?

I had my life all planned out, but God had other ideas. Life's not always fair—but God is. He understands what you're going through, and he has plans for your future. Good ones.

**LET'S PRAY:** Father God, forgive me for the times I allow panic to take away my peace. I don't understand why I have to go through this—but you do. And you promise to bring good out of it. Amen.

*"For I know the plans I have for you," declares the LORD, "plans to prosper you and not to harm you, plans to give you hope and a future."*

JEREMIAH 29:11

# 90

## New Relationship

READ: *Acts 9:1-19*

Saul of Tarsus hated Christians. He launched an attack on the early church with a determination and ruthlessness that brought fear to every person. People died at his command. Yet one day all that changed. Saul the persecutor became Paul the apostle. What caused this amazing transformation?

Paul met the risen Lord Jesus.

I hadn't killed anyone or tried to destroy a church. In fact, as a teenager, I attended church several times a week. I played the organ in Sunday school, and at the age of fifteen I became deputy church organist. I taught a weekly class of eight- and nine-year-olds about the Bible, and I ran a junior choir. Other members of the church saw me as a "good kid." Yet my parents had a different view. Internally, my mind roiled with rebellion. I couldn't wait to get away from home and live my own life, away from the restraints and tough love of my parents.

At the age of eighteen, I traveled by train from my home in Rhodesia (now Zimbabwe) to become a student nurse at the now famous Groote Schuur Hospital in Cape Town, South Africa. I longed to make friends and attend parties and concerts without having to report to my father.

My first Sunday off duty, I went along to the Mowbray Presbyterian Church because I had nothing else to do. The minister, Rev. Douglas Crawford, and his wife, Rhoda, befriended me, and I spent many days and nights with them and their two young children.

One Sunday I attended an evening service. Shortly after Rev. Crawford started his sermon, I sat forward on the pew. He was talking about me. As he spoke, I realized that not only did he think I wasn't a Christian, he didn't think I'd be going to heaven. My old rage took over, and I prepared to storm from the church, never to return. Fortunately, I listened to his closing words: "If you feel that the Lord has been speaking to you tonight, please ask me for a commitment card at the door of the church."

I didn't for one moment think *the Lord* had been speaking to me—but the minister sure had. I decided to take one of those cards just so I had something to base my argument on when I resigned from the church. But the flash of surprise on Rev. Crawford's face when he handed me a card at the door caused me a moment of doubt. Maybe he hadn't been talking to me after all.

I returned to my room at the nurses' home and sat down to read the card. It seemed simple. As simple as A-B-C. I read through the points.

*A* stood for **accept**. Did I accept that Jesus was the Son of God? Well, of course I did.

*B* represented **believe**. Did I believe that Jesus had died for me? That seemed a bit much, but I continued to read. "John 3:16 says, 'God so loved the world that he gave his one and only Son, that whoever believes in him shall not perish but have eternal life.'" The writer suggested I personalize the text by substituting my own name. Now it read, "God so loved you, Shirley, that he gave his one and only Son, that if you believe in him you will not perish but have eternal life." My heart quickened its beat. Could this be true? Had Jesus really died for *me*? Was he really offering me eternal life? I read on, more eagerly this time.

*C* stood for **confess** (confess the truth). The card said I should confess that Jesus is Lord and accept him as my Savior. This all sounded too easy—yet I longed for it to be true.

I slipped to my knees, rested my hands on the bed, and read the prayer on the card out loud. I went on to talk to Jesus as if he were in the room with me. Happiness flooded in, and I felt my rage fade away.

Something happened to me that night. No, not something . . . Someone. I made a new friend. I couldn't see him but I knew he was real. And it didn't matter what happened to me, one day I would go to be with him for eternity. In the Bible, Jesus refers to this experience as being "born again of the Spirit."

At the beginning of this book we looked at eagles. There's only one way to be an eagle, and that's to be born an eagle. We cannot become one, no matter how hard we try. Nor can we make ourselves Christians by trying to be good. We have to be reborn as Christians. And it's as simple as A-B-C . . .

- When, if ever, did you **accept** Jesus as the Son of God?
- Do you truly **believe** he died for you? Try substituting your name in John 3:16 as I did above.
- Where were you when you **confessed**—accepted the truth— that Jesus is your Lord and Savior?

One day each of us will die. Please God, not from cancer. But because of that decision as a teenager, I know when I reach the end of my life, I will step from my physical body into a spiritual one. Like Paul, I can say that then I will be "at home with the Lord" (2 Cor. 5:8). It is my sincere prayer that this will be your experience too. Pray this prayer with me?

LET'S PRAY: Lord God, forgive me for the many times I try to live without you. Jesus, I accept that you are God's Son, and I believe you died for me. Please come into my life in a new way, and help me to use this experience of cancer to draw closer to you, spiritually and physically. Renew my strength, Lord Jesus, and assure me of eternal life. Amen.

*If you declare with your mouth, "Jesus is Lord," and believe in your heart that God raised him from the dead, you will be saved. For it is with your heart that you believe and are justified, and it is with your mouth that you profess your faith and are saved.*

ROMANS 10:9–10

# Finale

## *Live like an Eagle*

When eaglets are ready to leave the aerie perched high on a rocky cliffside, the mother puts her head under one of her babies and gently pushes it close to the edge of the nest. Suddenly she gives a shove. The eaglet topples out of the nest and falls down the face of the cliff. Before the little one reaches the ground, mother eagle swoops underneath and catches it on her back. She soars back to the aerie and returns her baby to the nest. *Safe!* However, before the baby has enough time to get too comfortable, mommy eagle is at it again. Down the baby goes, followed by the ever-vigilant mother. Again the baby is caught and delivered back home.

Some time later, the mother eagle starts to take apart the nest. She throws out the soft feathers that have kept the babies warm. She removes the dead leaves. Then she starts to pull out some of the twigs. The nest gets more and more uncomfortable until the babies probably wish there was a way to leave home.

And, of course, there is. Back over the edge they go, until in desperation they start to copy the way their mother uses her wings. They wave them up and down, at first to no avail. Then one glorious day they feel themselves lift. They're no longer falling. They've learned to do what eagles are meant to do—fly.

As Christians, we are meant to fly. We can be quick to blame Satan when things go wrong in our lives, and certainly he does often stir up trouble. But sometimes God may be stirring up things in our lives. He sees us getting too comfortable, putting our trust in riches, our homes, or other people, and he knows it's not good for us.

There are times when we find ourselves pitching downward, out of control. Yet God is always nearby and will catch us before we hit the bottom. He wants to teach us to fly.

My prayer for each one of us is that we will start to copy the eagle—that we will spread our wings. That we will allow the winds of the Spirit to lift us above the pain and confusion of cancer. That we will be able to climb above the dark valley and upward into the heavens. Then, and only then, will we soar on wings as eagles. We'll have learned to fly. Our strength will be renewed.

*But those who trust in the Lord for help will find their strength renewed. They will rise on wings like eagles.*

ISAIAH 40:31

# Appendix 1

# Helpful Scriptures

Here are some Scriptures you may want to keep readily available. Use them in whatever way you find helpful. First, here are a few examples of ways you can use them:

1. **Meditate on the words and apply them to your situation.** "The eternal God is your refuge, and underneath are the everlasting arms" (Deut. 33:27). God is eternal. *How does that affect me?* God is my refuge. *What is a refuge? How can this work for me?* His arms are underneath me. So if I let go, he'll be there to catch me. *What does this mean for me today?*

2. **Choose one passage and personalize the words, then repeat them aloud throughout the day.** "Do not be anxious about anything, but in every situation, by prayer and petition, with thanksgiving, present your requests to God" (Phil. 4:6). [Your name], do not be anxious about anything . . . present your requests to God with thanksgiving.

3. **Pray the Scripture, changing the words where necessary.** "Be strong and courageous. Do not be afraid or terrified because of

them, for the LORD your God goes with you; he will never leave you nor forsake you" (Deut. 31:6). *Lord, help me to be strong and courageous. Stop me from being afraid or terrified of cancer. Remind me that you, my Lord God, are with me. Help me to remember that you will never leave me nor forsake me. Amen.*

## The Lord Is My God

"The LORD will watch over your coming and going both now and forevermore" (Ps. 121:8).

"He who began a good work in you will carry it on to completion until the day of Christ Jesus" (Phil. 1:6).

"And we know that in all things God works for the good of those who love him" (Rom. 8:28).

"For this God is our God for ever and ever; he will be our guide even to the end" (Ps. 48:14).

"But thanks be to God! He gives us the victory through our Lord Jesus Christ" (1 Cor. 15:57).

"And my God will meet all your needs according to the riches of his glory in Christ Jesus" (Phil. 4:19).

"He knows the way that I take; when he has tested me, I will come forth as gold" (Job 23:10).

"Fixing our eyes on Jesus, the pioneer and perfecter of our faith" (Heb. 12:2).

"Do not fear, for I have redeemed you; I have summoned you by name; you are mine" (Isa. 43:1).

## He Grants Me Peace

"And the peace of God, which transcends all understanding, will guard your hearts and your minds in Christ Jesus" (Phil. 4:7).

"Let the beloved of the LORD rest secure in him, for he shields him all day long, and the one the LORD loves rests between his shoulders" (Deut. 33:12).

"You will keep in perfect peace those whose minds are steadfast, because they trust in you" (Isa. 26:3).

"Be still, and know that I am God" (Ps. 46:10).

"But seek his kingdom, and these things will be given to you as well" (Luke 12:31).

### Joy Is an Action

"A cheerful heart is good medicine" (Prov. 17:22).

"Give thanks to the LORD, for he is good. His love endures forever" (Ps. 136:1).

"Give thanks in all circumstances; for this is God's will for you in Christ Jesus" (1 Thess. 5:18).

"Take delight in the LORD, and he will give you the desires of your heart" (Ps. 37:4).

"Praise the LORD, my soul, and forget not all his benefits" (Ps. 103:2).

"He will yet fill your mouth with laughter and your lips with shouts of joy" (Job 8:21).

### Strength in Strange Ways

"This is what the Sovereign LORD, the Holy One of Israel, says: 'In repentance and rest is your salvation, in quietness and trust is your strength'" (Isa. 30:15).

"'My grace is sufficient for you, for my power is made perfect in weakness.' Therefore I will boast all the more gladly about my weaknesses, so that Christ's power may rest on me" (2 Cor. 12:9).

"Those who hope in the Lord will renew their strength. They will soar on wings like eagles; they will run and not grow weary, they will walk and not be faint" (Isa. 40:31).

"Blessed are those who dwell in your house. . . . They go from strength to strength" (Ps. 84:4, 7).

"He gives strength to the weary and increases the power of the weak" (Isa. 40:29).

"Be strong and courageous. Do not be afraid or terrified because of them, for the Lord your God goes with you; he will never leave you nor forsake you" (Deut. 31:6).

## Words of Encouragement

"Therefore we do not lose heart. Though outwardly we are wasting away, yet inwardly we are being renewed day by day" (2 Cor. 4:16).

"Trust in the Lord with all your heart and lean not on your own understanding" (Prov. 3:5).

"Let the one who walks in the dark, who has no light, trust in the name of the Lord and rely on their God" (Isa. 50:10).

"The Lord is good, a refuge in times of trouble. He cares for those who trust in him" (Nah. 1:7).

"Wait for the Lord; be strong and take heart and wait for the Lord" (Ps. 27:14).

"So we fix our eyes not on what is seen, but on what is unseen, since what is seen is temporary, but what is unseen is eternal" (2 Cor. 4:18).

"But as for me, I will always have hope; I will praise you more and more" (Ps. 71:14).

"The Lord himself goes before you and will be with you; he will never leave you nor forsake you. Do not be afraid; do not be discouraged" (Deut. 31:8).

## Help Me, Lord!

"Hear my prayer, LORD; let my cry for help come to you" (Ps. 102:1).

"Though I walk in the midst of trouble, you preserve my life; you stretch out your hand . . . ; with your right hand you save me" (Ps. 138:7).

"The eternal God is your refuge, and underneath are the everlasting arms" (Deut. 33:27).

"Help me, LORD my God; save me according to your unfailing love" (Ps. 109:26).

"Even though I walk through the darkest valley, I will fear no evil, for you are with me; your rod and your staff, they comfort me" (Ps. 23:4).

"God is our refuge and strength, an ever-present help in trouble" (Ps. 46:1).

"Do not be anxious about anything, but in every situation, by prayer and petition, with thanksgiving, present your requests to God" (Phil. 4:6).

# Appendix 2

# Recommended Reading

These books do not tell you what you should be doing or could have done. You'll get enough of that from doctors and friends. These are light reading, yet informative and encouraging.

Broaddus, Jeanet R. *Ointment Poured Forth: When Cancer Fails.* Life goes on after the diagnosis. Cancer doesn't have the last word.

Buchanan, Sue. *The Bigger the Hair, the Closer to God: Unleashing the Cute, Witty, Delightful, Intelligent, Passionate.* A message of hope, survival, and God's faithfulness, in which the author encourages her readers to take hold of their thinking and move on to a more enriched life.

Cohen, Deborah. *Just Get Me Through This! A Practical Guide to Coping with Breast Cancer.* A practical guide to help breast cancer patients and survivors cope with the physical and emotional aspects of the disease.

Eibb, Lyn. *When God and Cancer Meet: True Stories of Hope and Healing.* This book contains powerful stories about cancer patients and their families who have been touched by God in miraculous ways.

Givler, Amy, MD. *Hope in the Face of Cancer: A Survival Guide for the Journey You Did Not Choose.* This combines medical advice and encouraging statistics about cancer survival. It offers guidance for the patient in regard to treatment choices and also includes a helpful appendix.

Hope, Lori. *Help Me Live: 20 Things People with Cancer Want You to Know.* Lori Hope seeks to answer the question, "What do I want you to tell me?" The author uses well-chosen anecdotes to provide sensitive insight into the words cancer patients and survivors long to hear.

Kaye, Ronnie. *Spinning Straw into Gold: Your Emotional Recovery from Breast Cancer.* This uplifting guidebook was written in 1991 yet is still around today. Through her personal story, this psychotherapist helps women deal with the emotional crisis of cancer and makes insightful suggestions toward recovery.

Silver, Julie K., MD. *What Helped Me Get Through: Cancer Survivors Share Wisdom and Hope.* Hundreds of survivors, including well-known personalities, share their practical suggestions and heartfelt reflections for getting through the cancer journey.

# Appendix 3

# Help Them to Help Us

Many times people want to be helpful. They try to encourage but fail dismally in their efforts. There are some words that a person journeying through cancer longs to hear; there are others they definitely don't want to hear.

I've asked around for suggestions from other survivors and added some of my own. Feel free to copy this list, cross out any that don't apply to you, add others that do, and pass it on to your friends and family. Let's help them to help us.

**I need to know**

- that you're here for me and always will be.
- about people who have survived cancer and/or treatment.
- that you are praying for me.
- you have hope for my future.
- I can speak openly and you won't condemn me for being negative.

**I don't want to know**

- about people you knew who died of cancer.
- why the treatment I'm on is wrong for me and I need to change.
- other people's horror stories.
- that I look awful, have lost weight, have no zest for living, etc.
- my percentage chance of survival.

**Please don't**

- preach at me—I feel bad enough already.
- tell me to stop feeling sorry for myself or to snap out of it.
- tell me to have faith in the Lord; that insinuates my faith is weak.
- criticize my doctors, treatment program, husband, children, or caregivers.
- tell me you know just how I feel—you don't.
- offer advice unless I ask for it (even then, be careful).

**A few other things I need you to know**

- Sometimes I'm anxious and can't explain why; I just need you to be there.
- I need to forget about my diagnosis sometimes and laugh.
- My moods change frequently—forgive me if I snap at you.
- I need you to listen to me and not be embarrassed if I cry.
- I am not my cancer; I am still me.

**Shirley Corder** is a registered nurse, pastor's wife, and cancer survivor (1997). She is contributing author to nine books and has had several hundred articles and devotions published internationally. She owns two websites: www.RiseandSoar.com, where she encourages and uplifts those who face a journey through cancer; and www. ShirleyCorder.com, where she inspires and motivates other writers. In 2004 she founded an online group for Christian writers of South Africa, which is still going strong.

Shirley and her husband, Rob, enjoy life in the beautiful seaside city of Port Elizabeth, South Africa. They have three married children and are grandparents to four special young people. Cancer changed Shirley's life, but she continues to use her experiences during her journey through breast cancer to encourage and inspire others.

# Meet Shirley Corder at

## www.riseandsoar.com

Find resources and encouragement.
Read her blog.
Sign up for news and updates.

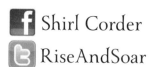

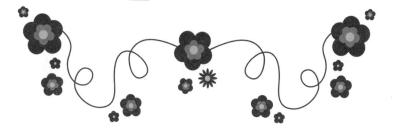
Shirl Corder
RiseAndSoar